BRIDGE OF HOPE

*The Life of
Rene M. Caisse,
Canada's Cancer Nurse,
&
The History of Essiac*

JAMES W. DEMERS

*To
the People
of
Bracebridge,
Ontario,
Canada
on the
occasion
of their
125th Anniversary*

PUBLISHED by
Bracebridge Publishing Inc.

BRIDGE OF HOPE, THE LIFE OF RENE M. CAISSE, CANADA'S CANCER NURSE, & THE HISTORY OF ESSIAC by James W. Demers, Copyright © 2000 owned by Bracebridge Publishing Inc., all rights reserved. Printed in Canada. No part of this book may be used or reproduced in any manner whatsoever without written permission except in the case of brief quotations embodied in critical articles and reviews. For information write to: *Bracebridge Publishing Inc., P.O. Box 23155, Ottawa, Ontario, Canada K2A 4E2.*

FIRST EDITION:
October 2003
10,000 copies

ISBN: 0-9682448-1-5

Bracebridge Publishing Inc.
P.O. Box 23155
Ottawa, Ontario
Canada K2A 4E2

Tel: (613) 729-9106
Fax: (613) 729-9555

ACKNOWLEDGEMENTS

Of the many memories accumulated in the writing of *Bridge of Hope*, none are more pleasant to relive than encounters with the people of Bracebridge who gave unhesitatingly in whatever capacity they could to the telling of this story. It is a story they live with each day of each season. That makes it theirs in a very real way. They shared it with unstinting generosity and consistent good humor. And so a very special thanks to: **Ken Veitch** for his relentless goodwill and direction, **Don McVittie** for his enthusiasm and good counsel, to both of them for making it possible to meet with the one and the only **Mary McPherson**. A very special thanks to Mary herself who provided the crowning touch to this process. I hope, Mary, you enjoy what you read here about your lifelong friend, Rene Caisse. Thanks also to **Mayor Scott Northmore** and the Bracebridge Town Council for not allowing us to feel like outsiders, to the staff at the Bracebridge Public Library, especially **Ruth Holtz** and **Nancy Summerley** whose diligence secured us the archival photos we needed, **Ted Phillips** and **Elene Freer** of Woodchester Villa who gave us such easy access even in off-season to the Rene M. Caisse Memorial Room, **Robert Boyer** for his heritage photographs, **Nicholas Roche** for use of his British Lion Hotel memorabilia, **Penney Obee**, for her ever-ready office services, **Wanda Cumberland** for allowing us to tour her bookstore 'attic'— the original barbershop of Joseph Caisse, **Paul Bennett** and **Chris** for their instant readiness to meet our photo needs, and Muskoka sculptor **Brenda Wainman Goulet** whose bronze and granite statue of Rene Caisse will forever stand at the first corner of Bracebridge as proof that this lovely story actually did happen in our time. Thanks also to the **Canadian College of Naturopathic Medicine**, Toronto, Ontario, through which this story will one day reach its long-awaited fulfillment. I would be remiss in not saying to **Philip Hannis** — thank you for the 'perfection- as- usual' of your artistic contribution. And last, meaning first, a warm and happy *sláinte* to my dear friend and peerless editor **Dr. Christine Jones** at the University of British Columbia.

— the Author

TABLE OF CONTENTS

Acknowledgments   iv

Part I	***Acts of Faith***	
Chapter One	The Endtimers	1
Chapter Two	An Ancient Dragon	15
Chapter Three	Unsung Aria	25
Chapter Four	Nocturne In Pain and Suffering	35
Chapter Five	Through Irish Lace	45
Chapter Six	A Prophet and A Lion	53
Chapter Seven	Cross the Bridge and Turn Left	61
Chapter Eight	The Art of Healing	71
Part II	***Acts of Hope***	
Chapter One	The Politics of Persistence	83
Chapter Two	When Owls Get The Vote	95
Chapter Three	The 'Forever' Nurse	105
Part III	***A Singular Act of Charity***	
Chapter One	The Green-Eyed Monster	123
Chapter Two	All About Yielding	129
Chapter Three	Yesterday	145
	Afterword	157
	Sources	161
	Index of Illustrations	164

PART I

ACTS OF FAITH

"Faith is, if not the most supreme virtue (charity is that), at least the most important, because it is the basis of all the others, including charity, and also because it is the rarest."

Charles de Foucauld

CHAPTER ONE

ENDTIMERS

In the waning days of the great boom they were called Endtimers. Like everyone else who staked their future on the unimaginably rich mineral deposits of the Precambrian Shield, they were, in the beginning, just dreamers. The discovery of the Miracle Mile, a surface vein of gold that ran as far as that, would make of Northern Ontario a veritable mother lode of endlessly optimistic prospectors and opportunists. The Lakeshore Mine at Kirkland Lake, the dream and achievement, against all odds, of one dreamer, Harry Oakes, was now the driving and thriving force of thousands of men, women and children who had better, more productive, hope-filled lives because one man refused to give up.

Countless dreamers had come, several prospered, many echoed the fate of their money, melting away one expired hope at a time. Gold, silver, iron ore, once just the guesswork of speculators, were now staked, claimed, mapped, and worked to inevitable exhaustion.

Miners who saw the end coming hired themselves out as

Endtimers, specializing in searching out the dying mines for any overlooked resources.

It was a quieter, less challenging task, free of the ambitions, jealousies, suspicions and subterfuge that had been the hallmark of the mining boom that once electrified Haileybury, New Liskeard, Cobalt, Rouen Noranda, Larder Lake, and Kirkland Lake in scrappier times.

In those days little could quell the riotous spirit of the region except maybe the forest fires that swept through on a regular basis. Townsfolk would race into the lake, wet blankets over their heads from the scorching heat of the forest fires and stand shoulder deep in the water while all that brief civilization of hotels, shops, mine shafts and huts were wiped from the map in a torrent of smoke and flames, a wrathful reminder to all the dreamers and schemers that there were four things they were forgetting, four last things - life, death, heaven and hell.

Of course, even without the fires, there were those who did not forget these things, those who valued not gold and silver so much as the little things in life, a peaceful heart and a healthy body.

While entrepreneurs studied the land for tell-tale signs of wealth, they accepted as a common enough occurrence the appearance of the Cree or Ojibway not known for their interest in wealth, moving in and out of the fringes of the white man's frenzy. 'The Indian', is how he was casually referred to, not with disrespect but rather with the reticence of the southerner who still was not certain if it was acceptable to know the first name of someone who lived in the trees. To most he might appear just another Indian in the endless succession of the people of yesterday who were known to have walked out of the bush now and then throughout all of the white man's years on this frontier, often at the most auspicious times, when a prospector or a surveyor from the more gentle climates was battling a debilitating frontier condition or disease, with words and gestures pointing out the tell-tale signs of life-giving leaves, stems, and veins of a specific humble stalk of greenery with miraculous roots that had permitted his ancestors to survive even glaciers.

Such an Indian was a reminder that only today could man be so arrogant as to think a machine could resolve the mystery of healing. The art of healing depends upon the healer. Throughout all of recorded time, men had become healers because they understood that the healer was first a human scanner who knew that trap lines carefully laid in the wild underbrush of the human heart, could recapture the runaway link needed to re-unite intellect to spirit, spirit to flesh and bone, that healing was an act of re-creation, the art of reconciling with nature.

As for the mystery of healing, science could no more isolate, dissect and label it anymore than it could discover a formula for the ceiling of the Sistine Chapel. The statue of David took its shape at the hand of Michelangelo, but no one would dare to attribute the mystery of its beauty to the sculptor. The mystery of beauty comes from elsewhere, from outside. The art of healing depends upon the hand of the healer. But the mystery of healing, too, comes from out there. The artist is the agent finding mystery a home. The healer takes the hand of the Creator and touches it once more to its creation.

There have been many such artists throughout history. A man of yesterday, an Indian who stepped into a circle of campfire light at the turn of the century would be remembered as one. A woman of today, a small town nurse by the name of Rene Caisse, would prove to be another. Though they would never meet, their lives would become inextricably linked and remain so for most of the Twentieth Century.

1922: The fires had come again. In the first week of October the entire region around the town of Cobalt had been obliterated. Ravaged in the inferno were no less than 16 townships. Nothing left but ash. The dead numbered fifty. Some survivors were living in old Toronto street cars shipped north in a less troubled time. It felt like the 'war to end all wars' had not actually ended.

The world was shrinking faster every day. Telephone and radio brought together what the war had torn asunder. Alexander Graham Bell had died in August. They buried him in his beloved Beinn Bhreagh, which meant 'beautiful mountain' in Gaelic. He was 75. That meant he was only 25 when he invented the telephone 50 years earlier. Instead of exploiting his invention, he surrendered his talents to the service of man and taught the deaf to speak.

Diseases had fewer places to hide. Medical mysteries were being solved. February of that year, a doctor who had returned from the War as an orthopedic surgeon, Frederick Banting, together with physiologist Charles H. Best, and biochemist James Bertram Collip, researching the internal secretions of the pancreas under the supervision of Dr. J.J.R. Macleod, had delivered to households worldwide a word languages everywhere were already learning to translate - insulin. Meanwhile, in a small town on the cusp of the Precambrian Shield, a young nurse was making sure there was enough 'cheap labor' to service her hospital wards and was learning how to organize it on twelve hour shifts.

The 'cheap labor' label would be a common enough jibe throughout all of the Twenties, ultimately culminating in a national survey that would report that the 'raison d'etre' of nursing schools was to provide 'cheap labor' for hospitals'.[1]

Was the age of 34 too young for a nurse to be appointed head nurse? Rene Caisse may have been enacting a little pioneering of her own when she accepted the appointment, the face of medicine in the early Twenties being still very much that of bearded professorial middle aged or older types, peering down from tribute portraits on this hospital corridor or that. They always spoke first, the doctor to the nurse, a token show of authority, of mastery of the workplace.

"Good morning..."

"Good morning Doctor..."

Or they spoke not at all. Some interpret authority that way.

Rene Caisse had assumed authority as head nurse of the Sisters of Providence Hospital in Haileybury, Ontario, as if it were a natural transition. Little changed in her demeanor or work habits. Life and death were still the daily, hourly concerns, the mundane details of hospital life her daily discipline. Exotic notions about healing bodies and souls were invariably punctured and dissolved by the demand of someone for a bedpan. Life, death, and a sense of humor were the triad of realities no nurse, for the sake of the life in her own soul, could ignore.

The obscurity of wards and corridors and operating rooms were the domain of the nurse at the beginning, middle and end of her career. Rene may have happily labored in that obscurity forever except for one accident of character, one of the many incidents of her personality that had earned her the responsibility of overseeing the nursing staff: she had a natural gift for registering the details of yesterday's suffering as well as those of today in the lives of those who came under her scrutiny.

So noticeably founded in moment by moment habits was her attention to the personal details of her patients that she was often accorded the highest accolade that can be paid any health care worker, she did not treat the disease, she treated the person. That attention to human detail was a prerequisite for greatness in bedside care giving, but it was not something that could be learned from a manual. A nurse either had the gift or she was bereft of it.

The sound of trickling water, a squeezed sponge in the hand of a nurse, a tin basin, and the soft murmur of small talk between the nurse holding the sponge and the woman being bathed is the healthy sound of morning in any hospital. It is the sound of renewed life no hospital ward can do without, the music of running water bringing life to tired ears, making them want to hear more, life to tired eyes, making them want to see its origin, life to the dry body, urging it to prove it is not tinder dry by releasing proof that life still flows within. It is instinctive in nurses to not muffle those early morning sounds in any hospital ward, for they rejuvenate and awaken rivulets of hope in the living and the dying.

The patient that was being bathed was a woman who was eighty years of age, under or over, maybe a bit. Like any body at that age, especially the body of a woman, this one was an encyclopedic record of the life it had lived. To Rene, at least, it was as natural to read a life from the signs and signals registered on and in a patient's body as it was for an Indian on the trap line to read the snows for the promise of bounty. She had the gift for reading patients like a catalogue, the past and present being mere prologue to ordering the prognosis. She could read old people the way Endtimers could read mines, and her speciality was in proving that the terminally ill have many resources left.

This particular patient had a gift also, to anyone who glanced her way the eyes looking back were a doorway to adventure. The elderly woman before her bore in her limbs and face the signposts of a rough and tumble life lived on the fringe of civilization. On her right breast was an ancient scar. With the bedside grace for reminiscence so common to the elderly, Mrs A., as Rene chose to make her known, told her story.

She had come from England thirty years earlier, in the early

1890's to join her husband who was prospecting in the northern gold rush wilderness. It was, at the time, so bereft of human population you could hear a human voice five miles away, the echo of a rifle shot traveling twenty miles and home again before fading amidst the sub tundra spruce and tamarack. Here the Cree lived along the rivers that ran to Hudson Bay, the Ojibway on the rivers that ran to Lake Superior. The white men who came here spent a lot of time trusting in their ability to earn for themselves heaven or hell, in this life and the next. But the Cree and the Ojibway had learned to trust nature the way the Northern Lights trust the sky.

Rene asked about the scar.

The flicker of an old campfire sparked in the story teller's eye. Ten years after arriving in the north, she and her husband had made camp far away from clinics and hospitals and the conveniences of the world, settling where the blackfly ruled unchallenged. A soreness in her right breast had lingered for some time and she began to suspect it might not go away. Gradually the breast had become swollen and painful enough for them to decide to leave camp and seek out help.

Before they could depart a human figure, a man familiar to the campsite from which he often came and went, a man seeming very much a part of the landscape itself, stepped into the circle of warmth the fire exhaled and made his presence felt in the quiet wordless way that was so unmistakably Ojibway. He may have been elderly, it was not certain, the Ojibway age faster, it seemed, than the Cree. He was calm, soft spoken as Ojibway men at another's campfire are accustomed to be. He announced without preamble that the woman had cancer.

The word itself could have put out the fire, so dreaded a word had it become. It had been feared in the shadow of the great pyramids, was a dreaded death sentence for workers building the great wall of China, had killed ancient kings. For thousands of years, it had been eating away at the human population of the planet. But in the 20th Century, the Century seemingly reserved by the Creator for the exposition of the worst in man, it was assaulting humanity with relentlessness, a faceless Windingo devouring its own.

The very sound of the word reduced the actual soreness to insignificance and, overwhelmed with melancholy, the woman collided head-on with instant grief, for cancer attacks the soul as well as the body.

As stunning as his announcement was, what the Ojibway said next was even more so. He could cure her.

In the stillness of the campfire, there came momentarily a willing suspension of disbelief, then campfire courtesies began to smoulder like green wood, yielding to the cold reality that 'cancer' meant 'Toronto' . In spite of the respect for Ojibway advice that both time and experience had firmly established on the frontier, the husband was determined to get his wife to that city far to the south. She had not chosen this life under the stars, trap lines instead of markets, rock veins instead of books, shadows instead of clocks. She had chosen him. He would now do his best for her.

They traveled south, train tracks rattling beneath, wheels crackling over spikes and ties with full trust in the navvies who lay them on the half frozen muskeg, the awesome prospect of cancer sitting between them like an in-law at gin rummy, weighing down their every moment, magnifying every discomfort, exaggerating every inconvenience. The worry and the rocking train began to work together until they were lulled into that humorless, wide awake world where everything is for the last time, everything is terminal.

Ahead still lay what frontier prospectors so avidly avoided, the city. Toronto was still Toronto The Good then. Or, so it was called by the people who owned her, ruled her, monopolized every opportunity in her, the white Anglo-Saxon establishment, who considered themselves good and had colonized more than half the world by believing they were the best. English or Scottish names had laid claim to the financial heart of what was to them still 'the colony', in spite of Confederation, in spite of immigration. Little patience was offered here to any of the recently arrived laboring class from Italy or worse still, Quebec, or worst of all, from Ireland. Not one chance in a million anything an Indian said would be given any credence.

At any rate, what the Indian said was soon lost amid the bustle of horse-drawn carriages, horse-drawn street cars, the nuisance of the bicyclists taunting the pull-horses with the arrogance of a blackfly, wheels picking up and carrying the sweet smell of manure in the streets, the hems of ladies' gowns heavy with mud as they struggled across unpaved streets with umbrellas and mammoth hats with crow feathers bobbing from the crown and everywhere shop windows with the ubiquitous big skirted Victorian gown on display, often pictured alongside the barrel wood stove that in the world out side the shop window every now and then sent up in flame some one or other Toronto debutante who twirled too close to the fire. And a piano near an open window enduring the touch of a student learning to play Greensleeves, a student with no talent who would grow old at the piano playing every song his mother knew, making them all sound like Greensleeves.

The gloom of the hospital corridor was palpable. When the Englishwoman from the north was told the prognosis, every gas light in the world could not have prevented the earth and all its wonders from appearing very dark. It was, as the Ojibway said, breast cancer. Advanced. The breast had to be removed at once. Immediately.

Such harsh words. Something about male doctors, perhaps. They could refer to any part of a woman's body and use words like 'at once', and 'immediately' as if the words had no edge to them, as if words could not slice through the very marrow of the soul, immediately and at once terminating for the patient the life that had been lived so far, so that, no matter for how short or for how long it lasted afterward, life would never be the same.

The Englishwoman weighed the options. A friend had died from breast surgery. Not only was it not the ultimate solution, it was not a guaranteed life saver.

In a moment that would effect the lives of many thousands to come in Toronto, in the far north, across the nation and beyond the borders of the known world to the people of nations not yet formed, the Englishwoman decided against the operation. The wilderness of the north had not yielded gold for their troubled pockets and the procedure was expensive. Fated to living one moment at a time, her death sentence even now networking its way through her breast, she slipped her arm into that of her grieving husband and walked back to the train station.

The return trip was like a tour of all the natural sights experienced in her lifetime that she would never see again. Fish jumping in the shallows below the trestles, a black bear cub chased by her mother from an embankment back into the shelter of the bush, the surprise rainstorm that gave a morse code reminder to the very marrow in the bones of precious long ago childhood and its many mythic battles lost and won.

The leafy forests of the south yielded to the needled forests of the low north, then to the barren stretches, here and there interrupted by spruce and tamarack, meaning nearness to the home campfire.

It was on the return trip, perhaps upon stepping down from the train or at the first whiff of campfire smoke that the Englishwoman determined to trust the Ojibway. After all, the Northern Lights had never promised anything they couldn't deliver. And the Ojibway said nothing about removing part of her anatomy.

Indians are accustomed to comebacks. It would be there in the Ojibway's eyes, the calm assurance that now the Englishwoman's husband would listen. Indians are accustomed to being disregarded first, then, the 'on second thought' ensnares the white man and he goes in search of whatever Indian had tweaked his conscience.

This Ojibway, like most, would have a voice as soft as the velvet of the leaves before him, a medicine man in full control of his audience. There were herbs growing wild, indigenous to the area, just a handful of the myriad leaves and stems and roots in a galaxy of acres stretching out to the frozen arctic.

Assigning portions, allotting boiling times, brewing times, steeping times, he demonstrated the recipe so that it would be hers to repeat, it belonging, like the leaves, to all those for whom the grass grows and the rivers flow.

One can almost hear that soft voice whispering across the century gone by, "Drink."

She drank.

He would watch her eyes lift from the cup, so that once again, onto the hope-filled eyes of a sufferer would be imprinted the proverbial 'elderly Indian with a natural herbal remedy'. Indians, too, had pride after all, in being remembered.

"Drink it daily," he had directed, calling it a holy drink that would purify her body and place it back in balance with the Great Spirit.

Then, his role among the white campers having been refreshed of face and purpose, the legend that the ever predictable white men feel compelled to spin about wise old Indians now having new momentum, he would, as expected and right on cue, fade back to where Indian medicine men come from, defying anyone to determine where. Nobody, after all, makes an exit like an 'elderly Indian with a natural herbal remedy'. Just ask one of them. If you can find them.

Rene Caisse attended to every word of the Englishwoman's tale with a stillness characteristic of a fertile mind. The nurse watched unmoving as the old woman's lips uttered the life-giving story. Any onlooker passing by might have thought that for the moment Rene Caisse had petrified or that her psyche had slipped into a brief catatonia. But in fact, her stillness was simply the hallmark 'moment of peace' exhibited so often by offspring of large families.

In a family of eleven children and two parents, a child cannot always find rest, peace, a moment of its own. With the comings and going of the words and thoughts and human actions of thirteen people, nature offers to the growing observant child a device for coping. It is a moment of stillness, on which on the very surface of the iris of the eyes the face of the universe is reflected, its message graphed into recognizable, comprehensible symbols, a moment when the intellect decelerates all other physical, emotional, spiritual momentum while the mind allows to be imprinted upon it a new learning.

Throughout the life lived by a child reared in a boisterous, unstoppable family of siblings and parents, that 'moment of peace' is mercifully repeatable whether in the midst of unfathomable chaos or alongside a softly murmuring stream. It is the moment of ultimate communication between the human mind, and nature, the great teacher.

Throughout Rene Caisse's life, at moments of great learning, or great trauma, the eyes would grow instantly still and a generous intellect would welcome onto its surface the writing hand of the great teacher of mankind.

As the Englishwoman finished her story, Caisse's still, respectful eye reflected the ancient face before her.

Did the Englishwoman drink it daily, the nurse would wonder looking at the ancient scar on the woman's breast?

Two decades had passed since the doctors in Toronto had demanded the sacrifice of a breast to the devouring death-dealing plague of the ages. Twenty years had been added to the Englishwoman's time on earth by the life giving herbs sorted and mixed by the Indian's hand.

CHAPTER TWO

AN ANCIENT DRAGON

Was it possible? A cure for cancer? So consistent with such stories of Indians with marvelous cures was the story of the Englishwoman, Rene would have found it not the least difficult to conclude that Heaven, when it decides to answer prayers of the critically ill, chooses an Indian to deliver the answer.

She was not predisposed in any way to disregard the story simply because its actual source was Indian. It was part of the heritage of North America, and part of her own growing up, that old Indians do step out of the forest and change the lives of white men. Childhood was flavored with legends of Ojibway or Cree intercessors imparting knowledge of herbal remedies to accomplish what white man's medicine could not. It was part of the whole of Indian lore that had drawn children into the mysteries of the old west for decades, and prompted many a European to become a child again and forsake the salons of London or Paris for the frontier.

One employed in the nursing profession, hearing such a story, might merely file the anecdote away in the corner of the mind, there to be eventually grown over and forgotten among accumulating anxieties of health care and the not infrequent stories of unusual if not miraculous cures rendered from time to time by elderly patients wanting to impart something to the world they are leaving.

Rene Caisse did not file it away. Hers was not that kind of mind. Nor did she compartmentalize it for future reference. Instead she thought it through all over again, detail by detail.

Out there, beyond the hospital windows, over the spruce, birch, tamarack, the red and white pines of Lake Temagami spreading southward toward the horizon, there were no longer any frontiers. Disease knows no frontier, only the need to find a shelter in the human body. What was this thing called cancer that feared homelessness so much it was ready to eat humans to make a room for itself? Was it a punishment of some kind, from out there, a scourging for man's pride? What was that song everyone was humming by that American songwriter, what was his name, Gershwin, yes. 'I'll Build A Stairway to Paradise'. Was cancer the whip with which haughty man was driven back down the Tower of Babel? Had something come down Gershwin's stairway, some invisible invader from beyond the Milky Way? No. Cancer had been around since Jacob's Ladder. And the Ladder wasn't Jacob's initiative. To believe in punishments on that scale is to forget that the Creator created out of love. Man, His greatest work, was in His image and likeness. When it suffered, He suffered. Cancer was not of Creation. It was of anti-Creation. It was no respecter of persons or of God in persons.

Far beyond the horizon, far to the south, Rene Caisse had loved ones, blood relatives and friends, every bit as vulnerable to the ancient disease as they were to the common cold that reinvented itself with each change of season. No one was safe. No one had the definitive blueprint for living a long life of perfect health. In her heart of hearts, as in that of any woman grown into the practice of medicinal arts, there lingered the yearning to be of use to those closest to home as well as to the stranger appearing morning after morning on corridor gurneys. The need to be of service to one's loved ones never fades. Rene's awareness of her opportunity to serve and her value to her loved ones had much to do with the blood lineage of which she was a product.

The Caisses who came to Canada in the 18th Century had quit the suburbs of Paris for the village of St. Agathe in La Belle Province, Quebec, still referred to by many as Lower Canada. Canada, then as now, was all about stairways to paradise for much of the world's dreamers. The family emblem was the dragon. Frizelda Potvin, Rene's mother, sprung from farming stock in La Prairie, Quebec, became a seamstress. The Potvin family resettled near Peterborough, Ontario, where Frizelda met her future husband, Joseph Caisse, a tobacconist, married him and moved to Bracebridge, Ontario. [1]

The newlyweds were compelled to experience a bit of frontier life first hand in their approach to the town, traveling the last stretch by boat, for the railway had not yet been completed. The rebellion in the West had not yet unified the country by rail; John A. Macdonald had not yet begun to count the railroad spikes needed to locate Louis Riel.

Like many young marrieds of their time, deeply in love with one another, with life, and with their new surroundings, they promptly set about to build a family of eleven children. Eight girls and three boys would be raised in the fear of the Lord in a town on a hill guarded by a fish-filled river.

There, Joseph built a store for himself, and one for his daughters who true to their heritage had discovered and pursued a career in millenary. Joseph, time would prove, had that precious parenting gift, the ability to dispense to all his offspring that rare ingredient of character - self-confidence.

Rene inherited the gift for imparting self-confidence to others with the same ease as did her sisters, when, adjusting a veil on a new hat for a store customer, the right word, the right silence, the right sigh, the right inhalation of breath would bolster the spirit of the client and send her away feeling refreshed, renewed, restyled, in fact. Fitting a client to a new spirit-lifting hat, as she saw her sisters do, was not a skill Rene forgot when she chose to top her own coif with a nurse's cap.

Joseph died at the age of sixty. Frizelda, a Red Cross activist during the Wars, would live to be ninety, a veteran community volunteer, participating fully in the activities emanating from St. Joseph's Roman Catholic Church in Bracebridge.[2]

Heritage such as this is not the kind to disregard the drive and life force of others, the experience and wisdom of the elderly nor take lightly life and death stories that had as a vital element a mysterious Indian medicine man. Rene's reaction to the story of the Englishwoman was predicated on every aspect of her inherited character. She listened. Listening, they say, is what transforms medicine from a science to an art.

Rene listened with an open fertile mind, all too well aware that doctors, when confronted with the unmistakable reality that the body of their patient is hosting a mutation of cells known as cancer, most often have to fight despair to remain a resourceful and comforting agent of health for their patients. It is not possible to run for cover. When it comes to cancer there is no place to run. No place to hide. It is the primary plague of industrialized civilization.

Rene wrote down the names of the herbs identified to the Englishwoman by the Ojibway medicine man, names scripted on the very iris of her eyes that fateful hour she listened by the Englishwoman's bedside, names of herbs that the Englishwoman believed had cured her of cancer.

How many scribbled notes had altered the course of history? Frederick Banting, on October 31, 1920, had jumped from his bed at 2 o'clock in the morning to scribble down, "Ligate pancreatic duct of dogs. Wait six or eight weeks. Remove residue and extract." And the rest, as they say, is medical history.[3]

Rene Caisse wrote down the instructions with precision and care, for beliefs rooted in pain must never be underestimated.

In the short span of twelve months, while the notes lay unattended in a drawer, the world changed. A new menace on earth was altering the horizon of lands one could never hope to see in this lifetime, the great monolith of Communism that had been raging tirelessly at the world out of Russia, was now threatening to devour a Europe crippled by post-war unemployment. Germany, hamstrung and disfigured all out of proportion to its cultural and political beginnings by the restrictions of the Versailles Peace Treaty, was in violent upheaval. There was a new Pope in Rome, Pius XI, once a librarian. Lenin wouldn't have to pay for any overdue books because Lenin was dying. The King of England was tired. Queen Mary kept an eye on the world for him from above her column of chin high pearl necklaces. Harry Oakes, the pioneer and dreamer whose determination, against all odds, had given work and hope to so many, was off on a world cruise looking for a wife. Remarkable voices now traveled by air. Radio brought hockey games right into the parlor. A broadcaster called Foster Hewitt had settled into a glass booth at rinkside in the Mutual Street Arena in Toronto and cried out 'He shoots. He scores!' for the first time over CFCA radio. Throughout it all, people felt pain and wondered why, grew sick and searched for health, were diagnosed and learned to live with death, died and left family and friends saying, "So young, so much left to live for."

Human nature had its own built-in defense against the death of a neighbor or friend or distant public figure. "They thought they would never die," people might say of teenage miners killed in a dynamite blast." Or, "So much to live for," of a middle-aged father struck by a train who left ten children behind. If a man died of a heart attack at 59 you would surely hear someone say, "In the prime of his life." Of another who succumbed to 'the old man's friend', pneumonia, at the age of eighty-four someone would surely say, "His sisters all lived to be ninety seven. He was the baby of the family, had years to go yet." And a man who died at 108 with eight congratulatory birthday cards from the King of England on his bedside stand might garner the comment, "One more year and his cards would have made a novena. He was too tired to wait I guess."

Amidst the bleak sorrow of a family or neighborhood death one could always be certain that voices would single themselves out above the grieving and utter a word or a phrase that for just a moment kept the dearly departed among the living, as if the death of a man was just the latest achievement of his character. In spite of a lifetime of monotonous evidence to the contrary, occasionally the dead would be discovered to have had a little bit of the Irish in them, that remarkable trait that allows his survivors to find him infinitely more interesting the moment he's dead.

It is in the wake of death that the living perform wonders and find ways to go walking in the garden with the departed.

Twelve months after the Englishwoman related her story, a voice raised itself above the turmoil of Rene's changing world to utter a phrase that was destined to bring the story springing to life once more.

He was an old friend, someone with whom she had once worked, an old man with a cane now, one of the many from among the ranks of doctors who would be attracted to her character and personality throughout her life.

The dynamic was a familiar one to her, ambling through the great outdoors, often in silence, side by side with a colleague, the crisp fresh air ever the reminder that in spite of what they saw and dealt with daily in the wards, life was a precious gift to be enjoyed to the fullest in the simplest of ways.

Vegetation grew close to his home, flowers under windows, greenery stemming the fenceposts, eight legged life populating the leaves and blossoms, wasps on the wing. Somewhere honey was being made. Now and then the gentleman at her side would stroke a leaf of greenery with his cane, stopping to look at its underside as if it was a patient in need of re-veining, sometimes affording it merely a cursory inspection and then after a swift diagnosis, passing on, satisfied, to the next.

At one point, several words pierced the pleasantry of the afternoon, and sent Rene's mind spiraling back a full year to another conversation about leaves and stems.

He lifted one particular leaf with his cane and held it there. She looked down at it.

"If people would only..." he began.

She waited for him to finish the thought.

Perhaps his reticence was born of the memories he had of retired doctors spinning fantastic yarns that had once enlivened his intern days of old.

Still, he once again raised and framed with his cane one specific plant.

Rene stared in silence at the leaf. Once again the eyes grew still, somewhere, at that moment, her siblings and their offspring and all the patients she had supervised in her nursing years were busy adding color and texture to their lives in untold activities, but right here, right now, the universe was talking directly to her. The veins and contour of the leaf were reflected on the iris of her eyes. She was startled, for a moment a trifle disbelieving. The plant the old doctor was holding up with his cane was one of the herbs the Indian had given the Englishwoman 20 years earlier.

"If people would only..." he had said, not needing to finish it. It was understood that anyone in Canada turning to nature, to herbal remedies, to traditional medicines for cures authorized prescriptions could not give would have to submit their expectations to the excruciating grind of the wheels of the medical establishment which could be guaranteed to grind considerably slower than the wheels of the gods themselves. This in a country whose founder, Jacques Cartier, had successfully cured scurvy with extracts of evergreen needles and bark in 1535.

"... there would be little cancer in the world," he added, finishing his thought at last.

At that moment Rene committed herself to an agenda, a promise to herself, personal, private, in secret. It was, put simply, an act of faith, the kind one makes while walking a country lane, pausing without planning to, the intellect selecting the exact intersection of sunlight and shadow for a moment of stillness in which to formulate a determination, or in a moment of arrested motion between the throwing of pebbles on the lakeshore. Or strolling in a friend's garden. If Rene was ever diagnosed with cancer, she decided, she would try the remedy this leaf signified. She would submit her own body as a laboratory for the testing of the Englishwoman's story. She would mine those leafy veins until she struck the mother lode of mysteries, that critical treasure, the cure for cancer, the combination to the lock that must be uncovered before cancer became an inevitable part of life to every man and woman born. She would prove whether or not she had in her possession at that moment, a miracle waiting to happen. Against all odds.

CHAPTER THREE

UNSUNG ARIA

Brockville, Ontario, 1923, world famous home of 'Pink Pills For Pale People'. The results of the tests were undeniable. Once more Dr. Fisher was compelled to raise himself from behind his desk and make the long walk down the corridor and tell a patient her life was essentially over.

It never got easy. There was no formula of words known to man to make any doctor feel comfortable at the moment of pronouncing them.

The dream of being a healer had never faded, never died. But moments like this carried with them an inescapable weight born of the failure of the medical world to increase by even one iota the chance of survival of the human race over cancer. In such a moment, memories of all the patients of all the years since a medical practitioner hung his degree on the wall of his first office might pass in review.

He would stand by the bed, waiting for his hand on hers to

awaken her. The eyes would open.

Mrs. Potvin...?

The sound of his voice bearing its fatal burden would tell the tale.

How long?

He would avoid her eye, something he seldom did. But this day...

Mireza...,

This time her unusual first name did not animate his mind the way it had on previous encounters.

A year?

He would not answer soon enough...

Six months?

He would stop rubbing her hand. Nod.

Six months.

A niece had to be told. Yes, he knew of her. Abstractedly he tried to recall the other unusual sounding name of Mireza's relative. Could someone tell her niece, get a message to her.

Of course.

She was a nurse. Her name was Rene Caisse.

Of course....!

Fisher was familiar with Rene. She had worked for him on previous occasions and he held her in high regard. He contacted her.

The message was, "Cancer of the stomach."

Here then was the old adversary taunting, torturing, daring. In the stillness that always accompanied news of a loved one, when the news was dire, Rene allowed it to imprint on her soul, the challenge of a lifetime.

Yes, she would come to Brockville. Death was stalking her family. The circle of life and death that was her professional life came now into perfect focus because her aunt Mireza lay dying on the banks of that great river that the early settlers called The Road To

God. It began and ended and began again, never ending, the Road always leading to and from the same beginning, the same end.

Scattering its length along the banks of the St. Lawrence, the town of Brockville was not unlike Bracebridge or many other provincial towns that harbored ambitions to someday be called a city. Long before people understood the liberation that comes from fleeing a city, children checked off population figures to see if their home town was getting anywhere closer to the 25,000 figure that would mean a new sign on the outskirts saying. 'Welcome to the City of...'

Brockville didn't have a welcoming sign of any kind yet. It was known as the Gateway to the Thousand Islands but not yet in roadside print. But it did have something world class and special. It had a theater with the largest stage of any theater in North America. Enrico Caruso sang there in his heyday. The town famous for Pink Pills For Pale People had made Brockville a place where millionaires could feel at ease with world celebrities. The strains of Caruso's incomparable Ave Maria could never be far from the mind and heart of anyone arriving on the main street of Brockville, passing the theater. His death had shaken the whole world. Italy, clamored to have his body returned. The Vatican paid tribute on his funeral day. The great ones were always revered as much in death as in life.

The death of Mireza Potvin would be a quiet affair for family and friends. Then memory of her would fade. Littleness in death does not make headlines. Survivors forget so they can beat loneliness. The loneliness of surviving was far from unfamiliar to Rene.

There was nothing known to medicine that would have any effect whatever in relieving Mireza's suffering. That fact was not spoken either by Rene Caisse or Dr. Fisher when they met upon her arrival. They both knew that years of research had still provided them with nowhere to turn.

The first visit to Mireza had been choreographed centuries ago when hospitals first came into being. First the management of smiles, then the management of tears, reducing them to a silent flow, then surrendering to the torrent that is unleashed when hands touch. Then tears silenced by non-syllabic utterances, then the management of words, until phrases could be wrung out. In them, resignation. In them, comfort. Then the silence of admission.

The science of medicine begins at such a moment, when the evidence in the sufferer is irrefutable and the medical practitioner determines how to proceed to bring ease to the victim. Were the doctor or nurse at that moment to determine to work solely with what is known then medicine becomes a craft in the hands of a craftsman. When the doctor or nurse considers the needs of the patient in the light of how much is not known about the disease and about the standard, accepted, available treatments, then medical care becomes science. The human touch of the doctor or nurse elevates that science into an art form.

It is key to understanding the mystery of Rene Caisse, to consider carefully the words of Dr. Frederick Banting:

"It is not within the power of the properly constructed human mind to be satisfied."

To be satisfied would be to accept that patients are not individuals, that their diseases behave in predictable ways, that the body and history of the patient have nothing new to bring to the battle with that disease. From all the evidence of Rene Caisse's modus operandi at bedside, the onlooker can be guaranteed that this was not her perception of health care. She seemed to instinctively regard each patient as an individual and unique victim of an equally individual and unique invasion of disease. It was as if each patient came to sickbed as a perfectly autonomous laboratory, housing within endless untapped alternatives to physical surrender. Dr. Fisher, it would turn out, shared the same view of the practice of medicine.

Both Rene and Dr. Fisher knew there were no known resources to apply to Mireza. Except one. She decided to propose to Fisher that they try the herbal medicine on her aunt. What did they have to lose?

It must have been an unusual moment when she sought him out to suggest it. What would Fisher have seen as she positioned herself before him, secured his full attention and then proceeded?

The woman before him would have revealed that curious, characteristic stillness in her eyes, the stillness that can be misinterpreted as judgmental, accompanied by an unusual and fixating silence. If eyes could ever be called silent, then, yes, at this moment, the woman before him had eyes filled with silence. Yet, in the minute play of light upon the interior eye, where the heart and souls are stitched to its lens, unsung arias were waiting in the wings.

She had a story to tell.

And so, Dr. Fisher, for the next while, warmed his soul at a campfire lit thirty years ago, a campfire that had found a way, through the Englishwoman and Rene Caisse, to never go out. In the story told by the nurse, the raw beauty of the country he loved so well reached inside and furnished anew his heart, making him welcome every word. The words floating to him down rivers and over lakes made gold by the Canadian sun's rising and setting and rising again, pine needles spitting out a last protest from the dying fire as night settled on the north, a midnight waft of smoked fish on a branch outside a tent opening, the curl of careers staked and lost on the mysteries of the north, some won, now and then some winning big, spiraling skyward from the smouldering ambitions of men's hearts and souls, skyward, ever skyward to the creator of herbs and dreams, veiled from view by the glorious northern lights hanging, shifting in the sky, repeating with every nuance of drifting violet and mauve and green, that where there are "Men of good will," there has always been the promise of "Peace."

Natural herbs, unpolluted by chemicals, pure, loaded with the high mineral content of the Precambrian Shield, had cured a woman of breast cancer. Could there possibly be any harm in trying?

No.

Perhaps no doctor's eye has ever been so watchful as Dr. Fisher's as he watched the nurse prepare for the first time 'the last resort'. Rene sought out and secured the herbs identified at the bedside of the Englishwoman one year earlier, sorted, measured them. Then, with the confidence of one accustomed to having prayers answered, she began, for the first time, to concoct the herbal medicine prescribed by the elderly Ojibway twenty years ago when Victoria was still Queen and there had not yet been a War big enough to be called a World War.

The experiment demanded complete detachment, total disinterest in all except the result, the self-abnegation, self-annihilation of the scientific process. So much was at stake! The risk was great and intensely personal. A highly respected nurse, well known in the region, was suggesting that a formula of wild herbs for which only she had the recipe could be the answer to cancer. Less sincere individuals would have given the back of their hand to the risk to their professional reputation. But the pages of history are turned one finger at a time.

As the first essence of the herbs rose from the steaming mix, a new war was launched, a war to the death, a war that had to be won, against all odds, the colonel-in-chief of all the allied forces of which was a diminutive 34 year old nurse from Bracebridge, Ontario.

Mireza had already spent tortured days and nights trying to organize the six months remaining, to set her affairs in order, to attempt to rush to closure all the precious initiatives of a life suddenly over. The duties of the dying, duties elevated far and beyond any duties of the living, are born of instinct, intuition alone the sole means to ensure that one is leaving behind the love that we are all called upon to will to our fellow man. It is the last chance of the living to give. In the midst of it, stepping up to her bedside and into those reveries made holy by the death sentence under which she was now fated to live her last days, her favorite nurse interrupted her labors. She held in her hands a cup and a ladle. Its fragrance was unlike anything she had encountered before. Not exactly pleasant. Not exactly unpleasant, just different. The ladle was extended to her lips.

She sipped. Not bitter exactly, but a deep wild taste like the unmistakable wildness in well done venison. The unblinking eyes of the nurse looking at her over the ladle held fast, Mireza reflected there for a moment of heart-stopping trauma, the stillness of a deer at the cocking of a Remington rifle. Sudden, startling, but not foreign at all, rather the stillness was familiar to the point of giving her peace, like the split second of life slapped into a breathless new born baby fresh from the womb. As if someone else was looking through Rene's eyes at her. This was no longer just a nurse at bedside. It was a face transformed, enriched by a hope it gave off. As if it had been blessed with a power not before known to humans.

What did they call those people who came from the woods, those Indians who knew special things? It was a word that meant a priest or something, a name for a human being empowered to be a mystical, magical, natural gateway between the known and the unknown.

Shaman? Yes, that was it. Mireza had just sipped herbal medicine from a shaman.

From the very first sip of the curious herbal formula, the six months had already begun to lengthen. Mireza could not have known that. Nor could she have been sure of it at any time during the next two months when she sipped the herbal formula. But much later, when the six months she had been given to live had stretched into twenty-one years, Mireza was able without doubt to trace her new life to that first sip of the formula brewed by her niece, Rene Caisse.

Could it be true? Dr. Fisher had much to consider. Had a cure for cancer come into his hospital through the person of this nurse from Bracebridge, Ontario? Could it be that a few humble plants in the Precambrian Shield were what mankind had been searching for since ancient times? Was the answer in nature all along?

Or was Mireza's cure a performance of super-nature? Was this a miracle from the hand of God in answer to devout prayers? Or was this a different kind of miracle, one planted by God in the sub tundra of Northern Ontario to end the chastisement of cancer on a civilization that had banished the Creator from its industrialized garden?

How would the medical profession view it? How would a doctor who had seen it all, heard it all in the cancer wards of Canada, react upon witnessing with his own eyes what men had dreamed of for millennia?

Fisher saw the cure take effect, saw the health of Mireza Potvin improve, saw her resume her life with the euphoria of one who has seen a death sentence overturned by a higher court.

What could he say to Rene Caisse? Would he acknowledge that the herbal medicine worked? Would he attach his name as a believer? What did the nurse expect from him?

The woman possessed qualities of nursing that set her uniquely apart from the public's all too familiar impressions of the nursing professional. She never accorded to any pill in her palm powers that the patient did not wish to accord it, powers that the patient, most often unconsciously, possessed within her own physiognomy and character. She was a living expression of the dictum, "There is no incurable disease. There are only incurable people." [1]

Fisher said the only thing he could say given the evidence.

He had ...another patient. Someone else believed. Rene had a colleague in faith.

CHAPTER FOUR

NOCTURNE IN PAIN & SUFFERING

The anatomy of a secret has as its backbone the need to protect. The Three Wise Men returned home by a different route to protect what they had discovered. The 'need to know' that is the media's justification for its excesses in this century once prompted history's most lethal despot to send assassins to Bethlehem, compelling a young woman with a secret to be led by a trustworthy man into the desert. Dr. Fisher had the trust of Rene Caisse. Ahead lay the desert of laboratory experimentation.

There was no escaping the bleak realities of being an innovator without establishment subsidy, they were there looking Rene right in the face each day when she returned home from nursing, because during those heady days working with Dr. Fisher and continually consulting with other interested doctors, the laboratory Rene was working out of was none other than her mother's basement. Now living on Parkside Drive in Toronto, she applied the herbal remedy to mice injected with carcinoma from humans. Here in makeshift surroundings that would have been instantly familiar to medical innovators the world over and throughout history, it was proven that the herbal medicine, after only nine days, would arrest the growth until it was no longer spreading into living tissue.

Dr. Fisher accepted that she was determined to keep proprietorial the herbal formula in which she now had total faith. Without knowing the identity of the individual botanicals, working simply with the herbal formula, he initiated a discovery process of identifying which chemical components could be taken non-invasive without adverse affects. Fisher discovered that eliminating the protein content of Nurse Caisse's herbal medicine would speed the effect of the concoction. By the process of elimination, the isolated contents that directly reduced the growth of the malignant mutating tumors were identified.

Rene maintained however, that the other botanicals were still necessary to take orally, this aspect of the treatment, serving to disperse and expel destroyed tissue and those infections, not inconsiderable, thrown off by the malignancy, the effect of the latter being to purify the blood.

It was a masterpiece of nature looking after its own. The stuff of which dreams are made, as complex a rhapsody of harmonious elements as Gershwin had imprinted into his Rhapsody in Blue that very year. It took Gershwin 30 days to compose his masterpiece, named "...in Blue.." after an inspiration by Whistler's painting 'Nocturne in Green and Red'.[1]

Ultimately, after those many months of experimentation, the day of critical testing arrived. A human patient had been chosen to test Nurse Caisse's herbal formula. The risks were so great. Rene did not doubt the treatment, but she had to determine that it would be administered without any unknowns affecting the result.

She was, "...scared to death," when she was introduced to the patient from Lyons, New York. The cancer had consumed his mouth and throat. He was listed as beyond any known help. The eyes of death itself studied her from behind the tortured face as she approached. Would the nurse reflected there cheat death of yet another early harvest?

Rene would proceed with the treatment once certain that all procedures were correct.

There followed a nervous few moments. The tongue began to swell. Had something gone wrong? Chills racked the entire body of the man, severe prolonged shaking seized his frame while his tongue swelled to a suffocating thickness, blocking off his air passage. Helpless, hopeless and hapless, the patient could only gasp for air.

"Depress the tongue..."

The doctor held the tongue down with a depressor until the patient could again inhale and exhale.

Seconds ticked by as the chills and the swelling threatened not only the life of the patient but of the potential cure. If the herbal treatment hastened the patient's death the hope for millions would be over.

They could only comfort him by doing the myriad little human things nurses do to lower the panic level of the patient, a touch, a grip, a circular rub with the palm, a word, a silence to share his suffering, then another word. For twenty minutes the fate of the herbal treatment hung in the balance.

Then the shivering began, almost imperceptibly at first, to subside; the tongue began ever so slowly to return to normal size. Ultimately the tongue depressor could be removed. Terror left the eyes of the man. Doubt left the minds of the doctors present. What they had witnessed, though they could not have known it, was the beginning of the death of cancer. The cancer ceased growing. The patient would return to Lyons, New York, to live four more years.[2]

In Dr. Fisher's willingness to respect Nurse Caisse's formula, we revisit the campfire of the Englishwoman. Mrs. A.'s willingness to warm herself at the campfire of her husband was born not so much out of her own faith in the extravagant promise of the Precambrian Shield, but out of respect, love for the prospector, her husband. Behind every great campfire is a generous heart.

But that mysterious wildfire so famous for wiping out the mining towns of the north with regularity was nothing compared to the wall of sensation soon traveling over telephone wires from doctor to doctor, nurse to nurse, victim to victim. A small town nurse was restoring the life force in burned out, hopeless cancer patients. Here was a classic instance of an Endtimer uncovering miles of miracles in cells overgrown with death-dealing mutations. Rene was inundated with requests for help from doctors who had no hope left for their patients.

She was asked to try the herbal treatment on one more cancer victim. She knew nothing of the case history of the 'other' patient.

She was told only that, "At the rate of the blood flow, he cannot possibly live for more than ten days."

She had not yet seen him. However, that intense silence, the deferential secrecy that settles outside a room where a unique patient is housed, marked the location where he awaited her. The man inside, whatever his degree of debilitation, had been singled out with great anticipation.

The door opened. The thick, unfiltered breath of death, heavy on the air, was almost impenetrable. Learning to walk into such a room was the most important discipline a young nurse could acquire.

Rene entered the room as nurses are trained to do, with a purposeful step, a function planned, a gesture projecting a service about to be performed, so that she would pierce the death smell of the room with the activity of hope.

She stopped. Seated before her was a man in physical, emotional and mental desperation. The features of his face had been eaten off by cancer. All that remained was tumescent, the blood flowing copiously, relentlessly over the mass. A man to make people screen their faces.

In years of seeing and hearing what cancer was capable of doing to the human body, Rene had seen nothing like this. The appeal of the old man was a silent one. Nothing needed to be said, his terrible presence in that quiet room needed nothing more .

As in witnessing a dreadful accident, the eye has to be forced, torn away from the object of horror. It is our instant reaction to the handicapped, first comes revulsion, then the empathy. Only when the handicapped recognizes that the observer has felt the first stab of revulsion, struggled with it and then overcome its effect, can the patient impart any true confidence in the person addressing him.

She turned away from the man with no face and began preparing the treatment. The need to be busy matched her need to assemble the botanicals with exact precision. The proportion of the botanicals one to the other was at the very core of the effectiveness of the herbal formula that resulted. It was a formula of proportions that she and only she knew. Even should some medical establishment stumble upon the identification of the herbs, their effectiveness would be mute without the exacting ratio of those specific botanicals. Then, when at last it was prepared, she turned to face the monstrous apparition awaiting.

Though nothing in medical reason could prompt her to expect

any positive reaction whatever in the face of such debilitation, she administered the herbal treatment. The success of the treatment on Mireza suddenly took on the quality of a fantasy. The suffering of the man was almost beyond endurance, his leaden despair clinging to the flesh, sizing the walls of the room, coating the skin, weighing down the uniformed, gathering like lifeless chalk dust under the fingernails. Was she trapped in some fanciful dream from which there was no escape?

She was working without a net, tip-toeing in the minefield of untried medicine. Would she wake up and discover herself labeled a quack, a charlatan. Would other nurses avoid her in the corridors of future hospitals?

So much for dreams of making the sick healthy. Getting married. Having children. Growing old. Living a life of honor and joy.

And what if it worked? Who would fall in love with a miracle worker? Would her life, if the treatment proved successful, be isolated, denied normalcy?

In the hours alone after treating the man with no face she weighed the options. Fisher had asked her to apply the herbal treatment to all his terminal patients. He could hardly ask anything else. The news was already being weighed and balanced by every doctor who heard of it. This was small town Ontario, Canada. Nothing could prevent a certain willingness to believe to grow into quiet pride, the kind that accorded fame. Or infamy. Was it worth the risk?

Time to go see.

Walk the corridor to the critical chamber where sat the man with no face.

Deep breath. Now, enter.

What awaited her inside the room was unmistakable proof that the unthinkable was taking place. The bleeding had stopped. The man was resting. He breathed more normally than at any time during the treatment. Right before the eyes of the medical profession, the nurse was, against all odds, beating cancer with her herbal formula.

Could it be actual? Suddenly, even in the face of proof, the whole series of events seemed surreal.

"I didn't think anyone would believe it," she said, and would say many times in the future. "It was so simple, I didn't think anyone would believe it."

The man with no face believed it.

What was in that herbal formula? Were the botanicals written down somewhere? Where did she assemble the herbs, there must be traces left over, fragments of the contents scattered on a counter top, dried to the surface of the inside of a pot, unusable portions thrown away into the refuse bin? Surely the botanicals could be identified from the left-overs.

Any doctor or nurse's assistant who had gone looking would have found nothing. It was not peculiar to the world of nursing that clean-up comes after preparation. The bachelor learns that life is much more manageable, much less susceptible to outside interference if the pots are done before dinner is served. The lark that would fly unfettered, disengages its wings from all strings in the nest.

Was this the miracle unfolding? Was this tragic apparition, this faceless despair, now restored to hope, evidence of supra-nature intervening mercifully in the affairs of men? So far she had been saved from having to test the formula on herself. Was she being saved for a greater purpose? Was it truly not peace that had been restored to the soul of the man imprisoned in a cage of malignancy? Did that not point the way, like a star of old, that promised peace to all men of good will, the poor as well as the rich, the meek as well as the powerful, the unloved as well as the loved? The promise was for 'all men'.

Once again that sudden moment of decision came, such as strikes when one is picking pebbles from the shore and suddenly one pebble feels so perfect to the touch it is not thrown into the waves but held, saved, stored in a favorite pocket where nothing is ever lost, ever forgotten. Once again Rene made a commitment that was personal, private, professionally secret. This seeming cure for cancer belonged not to doctors, nor the medical establishment, institutions, foundations or business interests. It belonged to all of mankind. Inside, deep within where vows are made, she determined that the formula would remain in her possession; that she would safeguard it against scoffers, quacks, the power mad, the Herods of this century and Herods not yet born. For the world that needed it so badly, she would be the sole custodian. Through her, the perennial victor would be cheated, through her, for the first time in recorded history, the victim would win. Against all odds.

The ten days the man with no face was given to live stretched to six months.[3] Other doctors, other patients came forward. Hopeless cases, debilitated beyond the limits of any doctor's capabilities, were referred to the Bracebridge, Ontario nurse. The results added other believers to the ranks.

In October of 1926, Rene Caisse was confronted with an appreciation of her work by eight practicing physicians.

Dr. R.N. Fisher (LRCP, MRCB), headed the list. Then came Dr. L.A. Blye (MB), Dr. E.T. Hoidge (MB, LRCP, MRCB), Dr. Charles H. Hair (MDCM), Dr.S. Moore (MDCM), Dr.H.T. Williams (MD), Dr. J.C. Robert (MB), Dr. J.A. McInnis (MD)..."[4]

They all...believe?

Yes.

They had watched her performance from afar, taking on challenges from which any other medical practitioner would have recoiled. She had thrown down the gauntlet and dueled with cancer without flinching. And she had won.

The doctors were insisting that this remarkable case not be buried and forgotten. They had determined to take action. Eight of them had signed and forwarded a letter to Ottawa's Department of National Health and Welfare.

Yes.

"To Whom It May Concern,

"We the undersigned believe the 'treatment for cancer' given by Nurse R.M. Caisse can do no harm and that it relieves pain, will reduce the enlargement and will prolong life in hopeless cases. To the best of our knowledge, she has not been given a case to treat until everything in medical and surgical science has been tried without effect and even then she was able to show remarkable beneficial results on those cases at that late stage.

"We would be interested to see her given an opportunity to prove her work in a large way. To the best of our knowledge she has treated all cases free of any charge and has been carrying on this work over the period of the past two years."[5]

They signed it?

Yes, all eight of them.

It was a poignant, sincere tribute from eight of the most respected medical practitioners in the province of Ontario who did not doubt that the elusive threshold to a world without cancer, if not reached, had at least been detected.

She was still so young. They were experienced and steeped in their profession. Yet science had come up empty. The formidable institutions and research centers had come up totally empty. Yet, here she stood, undeniable proof before her that she had presented them with an indisputable fait accompli, a medical marvel. Dr. Fisher's incurable patients were being cured. In each and every one the results were convincing.

Pride could be taken, justifiably, if privately, not in her performance but in those well-known names. Gratitude could be expressed, secretly in the heart, for the confidence Frizelda and Joseph had instilled in her toward nursing. Pleasure, too, could be taken in the warmth and encouragement of those brothers and sisters with whom she shared that heritage of self-confidence.

Once she had remarked in admiration of her family: "These are the kind of people that I belonged to, my home was a happy and a Christian home, where the love and respect of our fellow man meant more to us than riches."

This mountaintop was reached without ever having set out to reach it. Thousands had dreamed of being the one to someday slice through the Gordion Knot of malignancy that had kept mankind mutated for millennia, of slaying the Medusa of cancer that had turned the living to stone. What could be more appropriate than it should come to the world through a family whose crest was a dragon?

Alas, instead of the medical establishment preparing to share her joy, it was setting out to have her arrested.

CHAPTER FIVE

THROUGH IRISH LACE

"Life is short, so is money."
Bertolt Brecht

Rene Caisse saw a new face in the mirror, one transfigured undeniably in her own perception of it by an aspect it was achieving that she had not foreseen nor sought. Celebrity.

The last thing she had expected upon assuming her nurses cap at graduation was that she would be talked about, her name whispered, acclaimed, disputed, denigrated, suspected, admired, sought after. But all those things were now part of her life.

While Dr. Fisher directed her in the experimentation on mice, her name had become public property. Rene Caisse, Bracebridge nurse, treating cancer with non-toxic herbs, plants growing wild in Northern Ontario in sufficient abundance to erase the suffering of cancer patients around the world.

Looking in the mirror she could hear the words she had repeated to doctors so many times: "The treatment goes to the seat of the trouble no matter what it is; whether internally or on the surface and gives to healthy cells the strength to resist the demands of the malignant cells for the substance upon which the malignancy thrives, thus causing recession of the malignant cells from the healthy cells which have become stronger." [1]

The treatment for cancer that was in her possession was indeed the stuff of which dreams are made. Yes, it meant more to mankind than riches. Perhaps the alteration in her features reflected not only the celebrity status that was growing about her name but the responsibility she so deeply felt. That the treatment must be protected from exploitation, from falling into the hands of marketeers who would see money first and the remedy last, was already a prime pre-occupation. She must keep secret the botanicals of the formula and the process. How? The treatment didn't even have a name. For two years she had been musing on what to call it. It had to be a name that indicated its uniqueness, separating it from any known treatment for cancer, a name that would be untouchable, out of reach of the medical establishment, meaning it could not refer to 'cancer' or to 'cure'. It must be a simple name, recognizable to the initiated, but protective of the content to those who were not.

It was there, right before her eyes, the name, had been right there all along, looking back at her from her nurse's uniform, from her name tag in the mirror, Rene Caisse. Reversed and reflected back at her it read from left to right, 'E-s-s-i-a-c.'

From that moment forward, the herbal remedy would carry a name that gave her exclusive rights to it, and stamp on it forever the copyright of the most determined nurse in North America.

The treatment worked. None who saw it could deny it. Cancer

patients were being cured, their health, if not totally restored at least buoyed up upon a new and vigorous hope. Everyone treated was benefitting from the herbal formula whose botanicals still remained known only to Rene Caisse.

Then Ottawa sent two doctors to arrest her.

The Department of Health and Welfare now made known their response to the petition of the eight doctors requesting that the treatment be given an opportunity to prove itself. The charge was to be, 'practicing medicine without a license'.

One of the doctors commissioned to make the arrest was Dr. W. C. Arnold. The task seemed easy enough, confront and apprehend a small town nurse treating cancer with a home-made remedy.

To Arnold's surprise, he did not discover an isolated, fixated pseudomedicine woman indulging her fantasies about being a doctor.

Instead Arnold came face to face with a confident woman with vibrant eyes that could suddenly fill with stillness. It was he, reflected in her confidant gaze, and not the nurse, who felt uncertainty. Granted, there was evidence in her eyes that the trauma of arrest was deeply shaking her heart and soul, but the demeanor she presented was so totally professional, matter-of-fact almost, that he soon found himself giving her the benefit of the doubt.

He understood now why the letter of petition to the Ministry of Health insisting on a thorough study of the treatment carried the names of some of the most prominent, well-known doctors in Toronto, eight of them in fact. Not only was the woman not a renegade, she was functioning solely at the invitation of those doctors, treating only patients sent to her by their referral, and was operating continually under their close observation.

Arnold watched the nurse watching him, then, as it is said of showdowns, he blinked first. He did what was unthinkable mere hours earlier and brought up the subject of her conducting her experimentations at the Christie Street Hospital Laboratories, pressing Rene Caisse, the woman he had been sent to arrest, to try her treatments on laboratory mice there under the direction of Dr. Norwich and Dr. Laced.

She accepted.

The experiments took place from 1928 through to 1930. There, treating mice inoculated with Rous Sarcoma, she kept the mice alive fifty-two days, a remarkable life span for infected rodents. But she went even further with another series of mice and kept them alive for seventy-two days.

Rene's mother, Frizelda, decided to move back to Bracebridge, Ontario. The option of accompanying her did not weigh seriously on Rene. Every doctor in the city, it appeared, wanted her to test her remedy on hopeless patients. The city and its facilities were necessary now to the advancement of Essiac. Rene sought out and secured living accommodation on Sherbourne Street in that part of Toronto to be made famous as Cabbagetown. There in her apartment, inundated with patients sent to her by eager doctors, she managed to aggravate the neighbors, the local Irish and other shift workers who, through what Hugh Garner called 'ubiquitous lace curtains', watched the flow of patients grow to thirty a day, marveling and sometimes complaining at all the traffic to and from the nurse's 'clinic'.

She was tired. Nursing shifts in the Thirties were 12 hour stretches of sheer unrelieved labor. Except for a two hour rest period and her free evenings she was severely limited in the amount of hours she could do research. The demands of proving that Essiac was worthy of medical establishment recognition could not be sidelined. She did not shy away from the decision she had to make - Rene Caisse quit nursing. The mathematics however did not add up. She did not charge for treatments, would not, never would in her whole life, and she was now without a nurse's earnings.

As Bertolt Brecht would say, "Life is short and so is money."

Soon, Rene found herself once more on the move, this time to the town of Peterborough, where long ago Frizelda Potvin and Joseph Caisse had met and married.

The much talked-about nurse had only settled in when a knock on the door at 8 o' clock in the morning brought her world to a stand still. A policeman from the College of Physicians and Surgeons stood at the threshold with a warrant for her arrest for malpractice.

What must he have thought when the woman before him reacted with a sudden and compelling stillness as he, the world outside and the papers in his hand, became registered in and reflected from eyes curiously and instantly expressionless. Was she seeing into the future as she beheld the man at the door? Is this what the years ahead would hold if she continued to care for cancer victims, the fear always of a door bell or a rap introducing law enforcement back into her life and threatening her career?

In her possession were letters from the Ministry of Health and the College of Physicians and Surgeons saying they would not interfere with her as long as she did not charge for her services. The value of those papers was evident now. They were apparently of no value at all if doorbells could ring unexpectedly at breakfast time any day of the year.

With disarming calm, she excused herself to go upstairs and dress for wherever he was taking her. While she was gone, the officer sat and read the letters from the Ministry.

She prepared herself for the worst, the fatigue of two years of labor overtaking her spirit, weighing it down. Composing herself for the ordeal to come, she descended the stairs.

He looked up into her determined eyes and surprised her.

"I am not going to issue this warrant," he said. "I am going back to talk to Dr. Noble, my chief. "

Dr. Noble was registrar of the College of Physicians and Surgeons.

Once the officer left, the panic that had flooded her, that she had been so adept at being able to conceal, came to full flood. The visitor had made a necessary point. She was totally vulnerable to outside official intervention. This could happen again. There were all too many faceless, presently nameless officials in the Ministry who had not met her whose knee-jerk reaction to news of her work would send arrest warrants to her door again and again. How much could she endure? What was she prepared to undergo to see her treatment recognized?

Within twenty four hours she had taken decisive action, writing to the Minister of Health, the honorable Dr. Rob, asking for a hearing. She immediately received a letter in return granting her a hearing on the following Monday at 2pm. Enough time intervened for her to contact the doctors who had sent her patients.

That Monday at 2pm, Rene Caisse was received at Queen's Park by Dr. Robb, the honorable Dr. B.T. McGee, Deputy Minister, and Dr. Cunningham of the Federal Department of National Health and Welfare. Far from welcoming to the hearing an isolated, nervous nurse, they saw her enter the room in the company of five doctors who had been sending her patients. With them were twelve of the patients themselves.

It was not the first time nor would it be the last that the nurse from Bracebridge, Ontario, would sit in the surroundings of officialdom and expose herself to the scrutiny of professionals who could make or break her. She presented her case. The doctors added their evidence. The patients, on view, waited. Some spoke.

Dr. Robb listened, appraised the evidence, weighing it carefully, delivered his summation. Rene Caisse would be allowed to carry on treating cancer sufferers with Essiac providing the patients came to her with their doctor's diagnosis and that she accept no fees for her services nor compensation for her herbal remedy.

She responded simply that it was her intention to prove that the Essiac treatment deserved recognition on its own merit by the medical profession.

Robb, in a statement revealing his personal respect for Rene Caisse, said that he recognized her as an independent researcher in a critical field and added that he admired her courage.

As she stepped out into the waning sunlight of University Avenue that day, she might well have said, "Yes, courage is all I have". The age called for courage. The world was reeling from the disorientation wrought by the Great War, the end of kingdoms and empires had been accomplished in her lifetime, forces known and unknown could annihilate whole nations. Imagine then what they could do to one single nurse. Well she might have felt as Bernard Malamud would say, "I did not know I had courage until I found out I had nothing else."[2]

Courage, yes, she had that in abundance. She had tracked down the formula for the herbal remedy, made well-researched adjustments, so far survived the pressure of the medical establishment and was now on her way to healing thousands of victims considered terminal because her character was as persistent, determined and relentless as cancer itself.

Granted the tiny figure looking down University Avenue was no push over. But neither was Time. How much would be allotted to her by the Master of Time to bring her herbal remedy to the world? Was it not noted that on the Precambrian Shield there was at that moment growing enough of the vital herbs to heal all of known humanity? But the mind of man was slow to accept. Toronto itself had not yet made the complete transition from gaslight to electrical power. Hospitals could not take full electric power for granted until 1929.

Thomas Alva Edison would blush at the snail's pace of adaptation to his great invention. Perhaps that was mankind's fate for not always acknowledging the source of light. Did not Edison himself, having been gifted by heaven with insight into one of the greatest inventions in human history, man-made light, not say that he believed there was no God? How could anyone relieved of darkness not want to acknowledge and thank a higher power? How could anyone stricken with cancer not discover prayer? Just as there might very well be no atheists in foxholes, there was also a meager supply of them in the cancer wards of the hemisphere.

"All things were made through Him and without Him was made nothing that has been made.." Rene Caisse read in her prayer book every Sunday. Standing on the steps of Queen's park, overlooking the capital city of the province which had been blessed with the cure for cancer, the thought could not have been far from her mind that she had been selected, culled from the herd, as it were, to midwife a natural remedy for cancer from created nature itself. Nature was the mother house wherein resided the cure for all the ills of the human body. If the medical profession could be brought to believe that, it would have its load considerably lightened.

Was she really the prophet of natural traditional medicines as some liked to say? She would have to resist the term, 'prophet'. It was pretentious and precocious. Then too there was that other aspect that she could not have escaped realizing, "A prophet is not without honor except in his own home."[3]

She could not have suspected that pivotal day in Toronto that she was about to receive a surprising message from the most unlikely place a prophet might expect, her home town of Bracebridge.

CHAPTER SIX

A PROPHET AND A LION

D r. Albert Bastedo knew the value of a dollar. He knew as well the mountains of millions that had gone into cancer research over the century. When he had fixed one dollar as the price of his bold offer the romance had begun between a small town and a favorite daughter.

The big city had already taken notice of her. The Toronto Star headline had read, 'Bracebridge Girl Makes Notable Discovery Against Cancer.' [1]

The writer, Roy Greenway, had effectively profiled the nurse whose name was circulating through cancer wards in the province. Public interest had been peaked. All of that was good. Very good. But with the public attention would come the controversy, the suspicions, the whispers that no one battling the plague of the ages should have to face alone.

Bastedo knew that in all his career of dealing with cancer sufferers, only recently had he seen a sufferer smile with that cherished hope that, after all the fears and dreads that followed diagnosis, precious life could be prolonged, God had seen to it. The Creator of minerals and soils and plants that grow in them had unveiled a new lease on life for bewildered mankind. And it had been placed for safekeeping, away from the greed and corruption of a voracious marketplace in the hands of an incorruptible nurse whom he was getting to know very well.

Fresh in his mind was the face of the patient he recently treated for cancer of the bowel. He had sent that patient to Nurse Caisse. To say that he was impressed with the result was to toy with understatement. It was more than convincing. It was a revelation.

He had read the article in the Star. He could see as could the most casual reader what the future would hold for Greenway's subject, celebrity, exploitation, adulation, vilification, all the attention the world had to offer. And what would all of that benefit his suffering patients?

In that elusive, indefinable way that decisions are made in the hidden archives of the heart, Bastedo had reached a determination that the nurse with the combination to the padlock on cancer would live and treat his patients not on some far away precipice above a media volcano but here, in Bracebridge, Ontario.

Bastedo, standing on Dominion Street, looking at the empty, uncared for, seemingly spent and exhausted British Lion Hotel, was about to do what many a prospector had done before. He was going to find new life in what seemed like merely a burnt out opportunity.

The famous old hotel stood lifeless as the abandoned mines littering the northern cusp of Harry Oakes' dream land. Long before it had been repossessed for unpaid taxes, it no doubt had housed many a dreamer heading for the fabled landscapes of Kirkland Lake and its fabulously promising Lakeshore Mine, the humped and rolling acreage of Haileybury, New Liskard, Rouen-Noranda. Now it appeared as all dreamers do when the hope is burned out of them, blank windowed, staring, expressionless. But life is a ferocious force; as long as there lingers a glimmer of hope, dreams, like campfires, can burst into flame even in the darkest hours. But he would need the Town Council of Bracebridge to make it happen.

A man does not know he possesses the powers of persuasion until either desperation or a dream discovers the talent in him. Yet what man, even the most persuasive, can have any confidence in that talent when the task at hand is to try to be convincing before that most impenetrable of institutions, the fortress which no man can ever be certain of breaching, the elected municipal council of small town Ontario?

This town council was the organizational heart of a town with a history of which it was proud, and a reputation that was enviable by any Canadian standard. The flow of life here had a unique flavor to it that was a natural outgrowth of its history.

Bracebridge retains the intimacy of towns built before industrialization made them all look alike. The rise and fall of the streets still follows the contours of the land, having been laid out before there were ploughs big enough to level hills and fill meadows.

It exudes the self-confidence of a town that has a unique purpose and a unique vantage point, which it does, its location capitalizing on its waterfall which marks the end of the navigable water on the Muskoka waterway. At first the waterway meant transportation and fishing. It soon meant power. Later it would mean big money recreation, which it still does today.

It has had an identity since the era of the French Revolution, being registered and designated 'Muskoka' in 1792 after an Indian Chief by that name. It was a hunting and trapping paradise when

Napoleon was fleeing Moscow. The Grand Trunk Railway chugged within site of the river for the first time in 1855.

It was already famous for fur trading when Lincoln got elected. The first white settlers set up camp the year the Linnean Society of London published Charles Darwin's theory on the Selection of Species in 1859.

By the time Picket made his fatal charge across the open fields of Gettysburg, July 3,1863, the north bound Washago colonization road was already two years old. By 1868 road and rail were bringing settlers from Ireland, Scotland and England to claim the 100 free acres of land being offered by the Free Grants and Homestead Act.

Lumber was the great demand of a country in a frenzy of building. Logs and tanbark were the commodity for which the town 110 miles north of Toronto was known by 1870. The romantic era of the steamboats plying the waterways of Muskoka would last from then until 1930.

It was already called a village in 1875, but had assumed the prerogatives of a town by 1889, complete with town council, who had to grapple with the success of their settlement. Bracebridge had become the center of commerce for the whole of the Muskoka region. The town has never lost its sense of purpose, and historical significance, and still exudes the self -confidence that comes from knowing you are the center of something vital.

The anatomy of a small town would be unreadable if one did not understand that in community politics the neck bone of the town councillor is connected to the thigh bone of every voter. Voters walk. They can walk in en masse when things are not going their way and walk out with the slightest provocation for the same reason.

Bastedo knew the Mayor. Mayor Richards knew of Bastedo's reputation for integrity, toil and loyalty to his patients. Bastedo knew the members of the Council. They all knew him. Trusting in these very ingredients, alas, has been the downfall of more than one stalwart citizen throughout history who has found himself standing before Town Council.

Bastedo approached the Council and stated his case. To any other Town Council, gathered around their municipal flame, the man before them might have appeared as just one more medicine man stepping into the campfire light with an idea for a cure for the ills of white man's society. But this Town Council was different. It knew the story, had seen the article in the Star, more importantly it had been dealing for quite some time now with the enthusiasm of its voters for what seemed to all to be indeed a remedy for the scourge of the century, in the possession of one of their very own, a nurse every one in town could say they knew.

The life of Rene Caisse and with it the story of Bracebridge, Ontario, may have been considerably different except for one factor - she was popular with the townspeople, who born and bred there on the banks of the Muskoka had that proprietorial sense that islanders are famous for, of who they were, how their history would be written and how a favorite daughter would be treated both by their contemporaries in and out of power and by the writers of history.

Indeed in many ways Bracebridge was an island, mercifully separated from the big city ways of Torontonians by slow trains and bad roads, yet totally in tune with outside events through that very considerable human traffic that gave their rivers and lakes its tourism luster, while being at the same time far enough away from the fray to be, in the ways that matter, unaffected by it. The kind of town where everybody knew the mayor well enough to know whether his enthusiasm for a particular point of view was sincere.

In this case, his Worship, Mayor Richards, was enthusiastic. The

Council shared and supported his enthusiasm.

Bastedo suggested that the Town Council rent the British Lions Hotel to Rene Caisse for a clinic and bring her back to Bracebridge to treat patients there, in their very midst, on Dominion Street. He suggested a lease value of $1.00 per month.

They accepted.

The voice on the distant end of the phone was not unexpected. Bastedo was a strong supporter and credited Rene with the recovery of his recent cancer patient. But what he had to say to her during this phone call was as remote from her imaginings as the tumbling waters of the Muskoka River had been throughout her tumultuous last days in Toronto.

The old British Lions Hotel.

Clinic of your own.

Mayor and Town council enthusiastic.

Approved.

One dollar a month.

Come home.

The journey home was made through a landscape transformed by the promise of the future. The rocky ridges, so emblematic of the approach to home, so unyielding in winter, spring and summer, had about them the aspect of medieval battlements which, once they closed their doors about her, would protect her from the oft hostile elements of the world outside.

The purity of the air, completely liberated from the industrial sins of the south, applied a crisp cosmetic to the skin, making it glow, lifting the face, planting crystal sparks in the eyes. The silver bridge braced resolutely over the tumbling Muskoka River at the entrance to town seemed to have been lowered just now to welcome her into the town's midst. For the short block up Manitoba Street from the bridge, the road surface seemed to dip in a gentle welcome. Then came the sharp turn to the left the gentle rise up to Dominion Street. There, waiting for her atop it, was the red brick keep of the once entitled British Lions Hotel that would soon house the mysterious fountain of healing, Essiac.

It was not lost on Rene as she disembarked for the first time and allowed the topography to register on her, that directly across the street was the town jail.

The Council brought furniture. So too did the Mayor. Friends, relatives, patients, carried in the very best their guesswork could provide, a cabinet that might make a file holder, a chair that was sturdy with good legs and a stout seat for even the broadest patient, a mattress that was good as new, never been slept on. Bed ends. Pots. Glasses. Cups. Bowls. A mirror. A calendar. Linen, fresh, crisp. Note paper. A pencil. Someone thought of flowers.

Five rooms to treat patients were outfitted. Then there was an office from which the well intentioned brick-a-brac of well wishers would have to be slowly edited out, secretly, gradually, so as not to offend anyone. A dispensary took shape, crude and ill-equipped at first but with lots of promise, then a reception room where arrivals could feel their pulse quicken at a warm welcome.

Rene's first welcoming staff was made up of a sister and two nieces. By the end of the summer, the sign was fastened to the door, 'Cancer Clinic'. The sign meant simply that she had indomitable faith that she could provide enough results on various cancers that would convince the Cancer Society to accept and approve her herbal formula.

"I'll save a cell for you," the jail keeper said to her.

But the sign 'Cancer Clinic' caused Rene no consternation.To control cancer growth and alleviate the pain of sufferers was what Rene knew she could do.

"If it does not cure cancer," she said in her calm unhurried way, "it will afford relief, if the patient has sufficient vitality remaining to enable him to respond to treatment." [2]

As for the word 'cure', she would wait for doctors and their patients to apply it.

CHAPTER SEVEN

CROSS THE BRIDGE AND TURN LEFT

There was no waiting. The sound of tires rolling over the southern approach to the river blanketed the entire season once word spread that the nurse everyone was talking about now had a clinic. The traffic had begun even before people knew where Bracebridge was on the map, the silver bridge spanning the river hyphenating despair from the hope that is usually only associated with prayer.

The bridge was the very icon of hope. The sight of it quickening the heart. How many patients, eyes closed to conceal their pain from those who were driving them to their last chance, opened their eyes at the words, 'There's the bridge'.

"Cross the bridge and turn left," someone would invariably say, for by September the destination was firmly mapped out in the imaginations of sons and daughters of suffering parents.

"Cross the bridge and turn left," a husband might mumble as his critically ill wife sat silent in the passenger seat.

"Cross the bridge and turn left," a mother with a listless pain-ridden daughter might say to her son at the controls.

The traveler crossing the bridge, turning left and ascending the incline to Dominion Street would have no difficulty identifying the clinic, not only because since, soon after opening, its red brick facade was known across the province to cancer victims who had never been to Bracebridge, but because it was the beginning and the end of the corridors of automobiles consuming every inch of the street, the clinic doorway being distinguishable from others on the street hidden as it was behind the crowd of arrivals standing shoulder to shoulder, eagerly awaiting entrance.

The rich and the not so rich, the poor and the indigent on that sidewalk all shared one common currency, hope. The black button eyes of a fox fur draped over the shoulders of an elegant pilgrim from Toronto might stare unseeing, unfeeling at the kerchief of a miner's wife from Coppercliff.

Scented water on the hands of a socialite from Rosedale might meet stiff resistance from the musty parka of a lineman from the CNR in Capreol.

A pilgrimage is a prayer in itself. Tears have no denomination. They are free, classless. The dialectic of pain is no respecter of nationality, borders, religious denomination, philosophy. Sable, mink, muskrat cannot cover pain any better than wool or cotton.

It cares not for age.

But one thing would be absolutely inarguable by the time Rene Caisse's ambition was fulfilled: the Chinese and the Italian might both lay claim to the invention of pasta; the spices of India might come from any number of impossible-to-visit mountain bound countries of the East; salt may or may not have been the cause of the rise and fall of Timbuktu; Ethiopia and Oman might both claim to be the home of the Queen of Sheba, but the cure for the world's greatest scourge came to the world not through a banking tower in New York, a Royal enclosure in England, an academy in Paris. The cure for cancer came from a humble Indian in the northern part of a province in Canada and would be proven before the eyes of the world in the town that was Caisse's home, Bracebridge, Ontario, Canada. No one who came to her in the throes of suffering would ever have to qualify for treatment by knowing anything about geography or philosophy or religion or royalty of kingdoms and empires fallen into dust. And as long as she had life in her, no single individual, no government ministry, no corporation would ever take that away from them. The door of her clinic on Dominion Street, just uphill and to the left of the bridge, would prove that hope is universal.

The magic and mystery of nursing as exemplified by Rene Caisse in the Dominion Street clinic was captured by an observer, Dr. Leo Roy, who would work with Caisse and Essiac and would write his own manual on cancer. It can be assumed that he took inspiration for his writings from watching her in action with cancer sufferers. He produced for the cancer sufferer the equivalent of modern day sound bites that offer perspective and hope. In them we hear the collected wisdom of the centuries of medical practitioners who, in every culture, have had to find meaning in the varieties of suffering that strike the onlooker and the victims as so meaningless. They are included here in their original simplicity, a veritable catalogue of common sense. As we hear them, we can imagine Rene Caisse moving from room to room administering to her patients.

The patient who wanted to understand the process of healing was the easiest to treat.

"Attitude is the first and most important step towards curing."[1]

Those angry at God for their condition were the most difficult.

The pilgrims sighing from pain-ridden bodies in Dominion Street shared the grim view of the future being weighed by millions in the Depression era dust bowl of the United States. Wall Street had failed. The capitalists who had made it happen and who had not yet seen fit to set world commerce upright and lend mankind a new lease on living, the children of Marx and Engels who, between the wars were ensuring that the suffering of Europe after the Great War would never end, the exploiters who bankrupted workers, impoverished farmers, reclaiming property and cementing monopolies across the world had no power over the hopeful huddled before the door on Dominion Street. The oppressors of mankind worldwide could not reduce in even the slightest way those people at the door because they had already all been made little by suffering.

"Cancer patients erect a false self to hide their malignant thoughts and feelings."[2]

From the very first day of operations, a trend developed that was noticeable to Rene immediately but would also be testified to emphatically by visiting doctors and specialists.

"All the patients," Rene noted, "would seem to throw off all their depressions, fears, distress, burdens and develop a new optimistic outlook on life. As pain decreased and disappeared they would become happy and talkative. My waiting room was the brightest spot in the clinic."[3]

Bitterness in life, about life, toward life, left little room for hope. Bitterness faded quickly on Dominion Street.

"Patients were happy to talk to visiting doctors, and would tell how distressed they were when they first came for treatments and how much relief from pain they had after a few treatments. They were no longer sick at heart."[4]

Always, it was the patient who was humble and accepting that healed the surest.

"Curing is based on reverence for life and reverence for nature."[5]

Prayer and faith doubled the effectiveness of any treatment.

"Faith in a power from above gives us our wisdom and healing abilities."[6]

Down hill from the clinic the rush and swirl of the river was a constant reminder that this was about nature, normal and abnormal. That within nature the Creator had sewn the very antidote for any aberration that might afflict it. Clearly, heaven found irony an effective teaching tool.

What did Rene think when she looked down at that street. She had no time to think. Within weeks of returning to Dominion Street she saw her faith in Essiac drawing to Bracebridge sufferers yearning for a dip in the waters of hope. Hopeless patients had always been her first priority. But she had never seen anything like this. The streets filled with petitioners, wheelchairs, litters. Patients often arrived in ambulances for their first treatment and, too ill to leave, even with help, had to be administered to right inside the vehicle.

Often times, perhaps when climbing into the back of an ambulance to inject some hope into a cancer sufferer, that one, all too present reality became just too hard to bear. There on her knees, the smell of death rising in her nostrils, she could not forget that there existed a determined and organized cancer 'business' raising enormous amounts of money, a veritable river of lucre, for cancer research. Vested interests would naturally be compelled to discredit and even to annihilate any inroads in cancer cures that did not come from within the foundations and institutes that comprised the cancer industry, even though decades of well-funded medical careers had produced absolutely nothing in terms of a cancer remedy.

She struggled through crowds who by their very presence were showing their willingness to expose their despair to public scrutiny. Often their spirits were broken or lame.

It was human nature as a whole that was ill, not just individual members.

"Cancer is a disease of civilization —the vindication of all the abuses we perpetrate on ourselves and what the abnormalities and hazards of chemicals of our environment and external world do to our bodies. Over many years, we each build our own cancer tombstone."[7]

"Feelings used as weapons against someone, or self, can be as toxic as exposure to a lethal physical agent."[8]

"Only positive healthy thoughts heal."[9]

"Let go of hurts of the past." [10]

Rene endured the touch of people reaching out to stroke her as she passed, pilgrims in search of a saint. A very real danger loomed - the sanctification of a process, as yet unproven and a person, also as yet unproven, by the patients and their loved ones. Always there remained the ever-present need to present only a professional caring touch, smile, word or phrase, so that none would go away with her name on their lips where instead prayers should be.

Sometimes after the fourth or fifth or sixth treatment they would start to arrive by car instead of ambulance and be assisted into the clinic. Then, soon after, they could enter without any help whatever.

"This was a happy event for them because many of them never hoped to even get out of bed again," Rene would recall, placing in bleak perspective the opposition of the medical establishment.[11]

Meanwhile the task at hand dealt with more human issues. The stress on marriages caused by cancer was immeasurable. None could escape the grief imposed by that condition. Patients often failed when unresponsive mates or spouses visited.

"Deadly emotions are definite causes of cancer."[12] .

"Cancer patients have usually lived in relationships that have had serious negative impacts on their lives." [13]

The hardened heart was the hardest case to treat. Irascible personalities demanding cures found their bodies resisting treatment.

"There is no incurable disease. There are masses of incurable people."[14]

"There is no cure for cancer. There never will be. There are only cures for people who have cancer."[15]

In many ways Rene had to educate a whole medical world that had strayed too far from the underlying understanding needed to attack cancer.

"There is no specific entity called 'cancer'. There are only people who have succumbed to the process which creates cancer cells...those whose bodies have lost the ability to neutralize and get rid of all the chemicals, poisons and carcinogens which damage cells."[16]

The innovative intellect of any patient determined much of the body's response.

"The mind controls all healing processes."[17]

It needed a whole new mind set.

"Cancer should not be explained and treated as if it were any other disease."[18]

Those who resisted embracing the whole, but wanted only instant solutions were disappointed.

Always, the question marks lingered. Did this nurse know what she was doing?

"What is not known ...assumes the semblance of being a mystery."[19]

As Dr. Roy said admiringly, "Rene Caisse, in treating thousands of cases had dispelled some of the mystery. Over the years she had observed that tumors initially grew larger after being treated instead of shrinking, as one might expect."[20]

The disease called for a revamping of all preconceived notions of the illness.

"Cancer cells are those whose membranes no longer block the absorption of environmental substances."[21]

"Cancer is a deficiency of many enzymes over many years. The lack of enzymes weakens abilities to resist and fight disease." [22]

Cancer victims who looked for their escape in the radiation room, were invariably buried with their distress intact.

"The incurable are those who give reverence to science and chemistry rather than to nature and the life within her."[23]

The most overlooked of all the body accretions was the most common culprit.

"The majority of cancer patients that fail to overcome..are those who pay too little attention to detoxification and elimination."[24]

Toxins kill.

"The toxins poison the muscle of the intestinal walls and impair the ability to contract and force out the fecal matter."[25]

"The most powerful destroyer of a person's defensive structure is a 'traumatic loss...' chemical psychological poisons accumulate and penetrate the cells..."[26]

"Total body cleansing and avoidance of harmful and unnatural substances is essential."[27]

"Our bodies periodically throw off their excesses of toxic wastes by means of a mucus flushing we call a cold. Our bodies burn up other toxic excesses by developing fevers."[28]

"The poison and the deprivation we subject our bodies to are the disease."[29]

"Total detoxification can relieve pain that even morphine

will not." [30]

"Possibly the most effective way to detoxify is by fasting."[31]

In everything Rene Caisse did the patient was involved in an interaction with the treatment and made to take an active part in the cure.

"You earned your illness. You have to earn you health. "[32]

The rewards were a sense of lost power over a worn out body restored.

"You do the curing. Special remedies, regimes, or doctors don't cure."[33]

Always the patient was encouraged to look inward.

"Our bodies know more about how to cure and eliminate disease than science, chemistry and healing professions will ever know. "[34]

And, of course, from cultures vanished and some still with us came the wisdom of the ages.

"Eat only when hungry.

"Don't eat if you're tired, exhausted, tense or hurried.

"Don't eat if you're angry, resentful, worried, upset.

"Don't eat when something is eating you." [35]

The first day of the cure was the beginning of a lifetime of awareness and active participation in body maintenance.

"The price we pay for assuming that we live in a safe world is our health and our lives."[36]

Essiac was nature itself crystalizing into a simple cup of herbal formula.

"The active and healing ingredients of herbs are the multitudes of enzymes their cells create." [37]

Always, the remedy was but the beginning of a new life, lived by new rules or the restoration of rules long ago discarded.

"Diseases are messengers from the soul demanding us

to...change."[38]

"Don't give in to temptations to go back to your old ways and excesses."[39]

"Stay away from spiteful, negative, irritating, overbearing, people. You don't need friends who find fault."[40]

"The magic key to cancer curing, to cancer prevention, is to live, to really live...full of the vigor and hope...to live every true vital force in you."[41] .

Rene could have been all but consumed by the demands of the world that had so quickly mushroomed around the Dominion Street clinic. But not too long after the clinic opening, the identity of a new cancer sufferer reaching her ear brought her into sharp focus.

Who?

Your mother.

CHAPTER EIGHT

THE ART OF HEALING

Frizelda Caisse was 72 years of age when Rene approached her sickbed. She had borne eleven children. The four doctors she had consulted had diagnosed gallstones. Unsatisfied, Rene had called the international specialist Dr. Roscoe Graham. He found cancer.

How long?

Days. It was in the liver.

Frizelda had been known to say with good humor that she would trade eight girls for one boy. But it was a daughter upon whose knowledge her health now depended.

The challenge before Rene was the most important of her life. In spite of all the cases successfully treated so far, what if...?

No time for what ifs! The crisis was made even more pointed by someone who had been opposed to Rene's work all along: Dr. McGibbon. He challenged her to cure her own mother.

Without telling Frizelda the content of Dr. Graham's diagnosis,

Rene began the treatments with the same precision for detail and the same cautious regard for the patient afforded many of the thousands of others who had and would come to the clinic.

She treated Frizelda for ten days, trying not to consider how much more important this patient was to her than all the others. There always seemed to be more women than men. Women were, after all, more in tune with their physical needs than were men. A woman did not need a husband to tell her she wasn't feeling well. She just set out to find a doctor and kept searching until he found the cause of her discomfort. Men needed to be told to trim their moustaches, shave the hair in their ears, cut their toenails. Women do not need men to tell them they are not looking their best. What husband ever said, 'Go buy some makeup'. Women know what they need to make them look better. That is the secret of the cosmetic empires all over the world. A little jar of this, a scent of that, and all your problems will fade away. A promise in a tube of lipstick. Power in a make-up compact. Hope in a powder puff.

Was Essiac a powder puff? Was it hope in cosmetic form? The definitive response can only come from the patient who had been treated successfully.

Ask Nellie McVittie. She was reduced to more than 86 pounds by the time she was carried into the clinic, so small she was almost not there, that mysterious invisibility cancer imposes on character and the history of its victims already shrouding her personality, the accomplishments of a lifetime, obliterating the names and faces of those she loved and those who loved her.

"Cancer is an emotionless, joy-deficiency disease," as Dr. Leo Roy would say. [1]

McVittie's physician in Sudbury, Dr. Dale, had diagnosed cancer of the neck of the womb, uterine cancer, the most dreaded words a woman could hear. In all the decades of research and all the millions of dollars gone into experimentation, all science could offer McVittie was to cauterize the neck of the womb, followed by radium treatments.

She was hemorrhaging when she arrived for the first treatment, unable to move about on her own. She felt almost immediate relief after the first Essiac treatment. McVittie stayed in Bracebridge two months taking regular treatments.

"Healing", as Dr. Leo Roy would say, "is not a casual pass time, nor a spectator sport. It is a function of personal responsibility and involvement." [2]

After eight weeks, McVittie returned to Sudbury, declaring, "Miss Caisse's treatment certainly put me back on my feet."

She was soon on her way back to a former weight of 107 pounds.

A powder puff hope? Ask Tony Bazuk.

Bazuk was a young Ukranian from the Ukrainian settlements in Manitoba who spoke what English he could hesitatingly but determinedly. He now worked as a CNR engine watchman out of Capreol. Having been stricken with lip cancer he went to London, Ontario, to receive radium treatment from a Dr. McNeil. After radium the lip swelled up so that Tony could see it over the tip of his nose. Back in Capreol, co-workers on the railroad raised money to send him to Bracebridge. When he arrived his face was disfigured to the extent that Rene found it difficult to look at him.

She applied some salve to his lip and treated him giving him instructions that he was to return in two weeks. He felt immediate relief after the first treatment. But when the two weeks passed, he was unable to return to Bracebridge on time. When he did return soon after, nothing remained of the lip cancer except a small scar from the radium treatment. In six months time he was back at work in Capreol with a new slogan for life: "Eat for one man, work for three, sleep like a baby."[3]

Powder puff hope? Ask May Henderson.

When Henderson arrived at the clinic she was a walking memory of Mrs. A., the Englishwoman whose story had started it all, who had been cured by an Indian walking out of the dark shadows at the edge of a long ago campfire. Henderson had tumors in both breasts and had been advised to have a double mastectomy. Only after being given this advice did she discover she also had tumors in the uterus.

She refused the surgery out of fear and complete lack of confidence in the outcome. She bore the telltale marks of the ravaging cancer, her skin a muddy yellow, thinning hair, blue eyes turned grey and stony, and she was hemorrhaging. Although Dr. J.A. McInnis advised Rene that treating Henderson would be useless, she began the treatments.

"Tumors are not body mistakes," Dr. Leo Roy would say. "Nature does not make mistakes. Tumors are body wisdom at work. Tumors are a warning that the body is super saturated with virulent toxins and poisons..something either damaged and poisoned or cut off circulation to and from this tissue and created conditions like a swamp."[4]

At first the lumps grew harder, then Henderson began to discharge 'great masses of fleshy material' as she would recall later. Within a few months Henderson had returned to work.

Powder puff hope? Ask the doctors who sent the hopeless cases to her. That was always Rene's answer. She had an endless supply of such doctors who watched in wonderment from afar as their suffering patients felt the touch of the Bracebridge nurse on their lives.

Some were unable to enter the clinic on their own power, but able to walk out upright after treatment. Always they came with doctor's referrals.

Gradually, Rene reduced her mother Frizelda's treatments to one a week. The cancer completely disappeared from the liver. Frizelda never knew she was being treated for cancer, would live eighteen more years and die at the age of ninety surrounded by grandchildren and great-grandchildren, totally happy that she had not traded in one particular daughter for a boy.

At her mother's death, at the age of 90, Rene was able to say that those intervening years were, "Eighteen years of life she would not have had without Essiac."

But then, "Healing is how you live your life." [5]

For almost eight years, thousands of patients, many of them considered hopeless, would be sent 'over the bridge' to the clinic on Dominion Street by their doctors after medical science had failed. Throughout those years Rene continued to believe that she would be able to accumulate enough proof of the effectiveness of Essiac that it would be recognized as a treatment for cancer.

The successes mounted. So did jealousies. They emanated without doubt from within the medical establishment. Caisse detected a slight change in some of the doctors who had been sending her patients when some patients began to show up at the clinic without referrals. She began to believe that doctors were being pressured, in spite of the successes, to distance themselves from Essiac herbal treatments. The sensation, the instinct, the intuition that, out there, forces were aligning themselves to deny Essiac recognition took root not in her heart or soul which remained generous and forgiving throughout the years of toil, but in the mind. It had a name, the dynamic that seemed to be at work, if not orchestrated, then at least consistent in its refusal to acknowledge the enthusiasm of individual doctors and the evidence of many thousands of cured patients. The word that emerged from all the evidence gathering on the horizon was one that, once it spelled itself out in her consciousness, was seldom ever to leave her thoughts.

Conspiracy.

Few locations in the North American hemisphere could dispel the sour suspicion of conspiracy like the corner of University and College Streets in Toronto. Famous worldwide as the location of the offices and laboratory of the most respected man in Canadian medicine, Dr. Frederick Banting, it was, if not a shrine to integrity and perseverance, at least an icon of scientific purity and all the credibility that that implies. His very name had become a primary source of pride throughout the whole world. In 1923, he had been awarded the Nobel Prize for medicine. His discovery of insulin pierced the shadowed world of 20th century sufferers and cast a glow that would for the balance of the century illuminate the gloom that so often besets the hard-pressed medical researcher.

Banting had been made aware of the nurse in the Twenties. At one point, Rene's decision to safeguard the treatment and her role in its usage by not charging for the treatment meant that she could not afford to live in Toronto. A decision had to be made. Protect her own health by taking a much needed paid nursing position or lose the ability to pilot her treatment successfully through the maze of medical establishment procedures for it to be recognized.

She had accepted a nursing post offered her in Timmins, Ontario, meaning she was returning to the North, close to Haileybury where the treatment first came to the world through the story of the Englishwoman. Once there she was soon exclusively treating the cancer patients of Dr. J. McInnis.

Here, indisputably, the treatment cured the bowel cancer of one of McInnis's patients. It was this cure that brought Essiac and Rene Caisse to the attention of Dr. Frederick Banting.

His conclusion that Essiac 'activated the pancreatic gland' thrilled and inspired the doctors treating cancer. Now, through the auspices of Dr. Faulkner, Minister of Health, she was on her way to see Banting.

Banting would easily have, at a glance, fulfilled everyone's expectations of what a world famous doctor and discoverer of insulin should look like. He had that pharmacist's or dentist's look of the well-scrubbed, austere student of medicines, his wire frame glasses windows onto a mind with encyclopedic knowledge of medical histories. Few men could have better understood the jealousies and intrigues of the medical establishment like Banting. He too had rebuked its pretensions in his own way. When the Nobel Prize was awarded to Macleod and Banting, he insisted it read Banting and Macleod for he considered Dr. J.J. MacLeod's contribution to the discovery of insulin as not as consequential as his own or as that of physiologist Dr. Charles H. Best. He insisted also in splitting his Prize with Best whom he considered the more important contributor to the process. Macleod for his part split his prize with biochemist James Bertram Collip, the fourth man on the team. The Nobel Prize meant $40,000. Splitting it, meant each one received $10,000 of the prize money. It was characteristic of Banting to share such a sum, he already having established a reputation of having very little regard for money. In fact, so uncaring was he about finances that his research after the awarding of the prize was threatened by the fact that he simply had no ability to raise it or make it. The Canadian government in honoring him for his discovery and rewarding him financially saved him from a struggle that would have been unavoidable given his attitude.

It was with confidence in the peer reception that she would receive that Caisse presented her scientific evidence there to the Department of Medical Research. Five doctors accompanied her when she went to a meeting with the famous discoverer of insulin. The reception was warm, the personal considerations between the two

Canadian icons of experimental medicine, immediately kind. There can be no doubt that an instantaneous rapport governed their exchange. Banting had read the case histories, studied the photographs and x-rays of patients.

"I will not say you have a cure for cancer. But you have more evidence of a beneficial treatment for cancer than anyone in the world."[6]

The words of his letter of July 23, 1936, guided her thoughts.

"You will not be asked to divulge any secret concerning your treatment. All experimental results must be submitted to me for my approval before being announced to anyone, including the newspapers or published in medical journals."[7]

Rene then heard words that any pioneer in medicine would well savor and cherish. He offered to share his laboratory in the Banting Institute with her.

Alas, added conditions, necessary for Banting, weighed heavily on Rene.

It would require her to apply to the University of Toronto for facilities and permission to do more extensive research. But it would mean Caisse would have to reveal to the authorities much of what she had so far successfully kept a secret.

"He also made it quite clear," she would so often recall, "I'd have to give up my clinic if I went to work with him."

In short it was back to mice. She had already worked on mice.

"I felt it was inhuman for them to ask me to give up treating patients while I showed them whether it would work on mice."

The prospect meant the formula disappearing into the files never to be returned, or falling under some ban that would prevent cancer patients from receiving it during the pre-authorization research.

The reaction on Dominion Street was immediate and loud.

"There was a big uproar about it because the patients were terrified I would leave them..."

The chance for Rene to work with Dr. Banting meant, to many of the doctors who had supported her throughout the years and sent her their patients, that they too would be working, through their case histories, with Banting. Many doctors said she should jump at the chance.

Caisse walked away from the Banting offer.

"It was an agonizing decision..."

She knew she could prove its worth in practical application on human sufferers, rather than wait years while millions of dollars funded researchers to make charts and graphs of what she already knew.

But she was, "...not going to let people die while I do it."

Nor did she intend to see the administering of the great discovery removed from her reach. She intended to pilot her own discoveries through what was to come.

Banting's offer would have given Rene the very thing that Banting himself had so badly needed at one time, laboratory access and more importantly, through the laboratory access, the hope of financial support somewhere in the future. The laboratory and the move to Toronto would have cost money. Without a salary from nursing and not accepting any money from her cancer patients for treatment (she had one time chased a patient down the street to return money he had left as compensation), she had to rely on friends and relatives for support. Much later she would reveal that these supporters who had been so instrumental in keeping her treatments alive, pressured her not to take the laboratory offer, saying they would no longer support her if she turned her formula over to those who would remove it from public use, then later, and most assuredly make a fortune from it.

In spite of her turning him down, Banting's faith in the nurse was evident by the degree of disappointment registered in his letter to her of August 11.

"I think you will regret that you have not availed yourself of the offer made by this laboratory. However, if at some future time you again decide to have the treatment investigated, I am sure that Dr. Faulkner and myself would reconsider the matter."[8]

From the windows of Dominion Street, she might many a time have questioned her refusal of Banting's offer.

"In a way," she said, "I have been sorry that I had to refuse it..."

But the rare luxury of having the time to look down at the cars crowding the shoulders of the street outside the clinic, downhill to the rushing river and the bridge carrying sufferers to and from her hillside of miracles, always restored her determination to be first a nurse to human suffering.

"...but I would still do the same thing again."

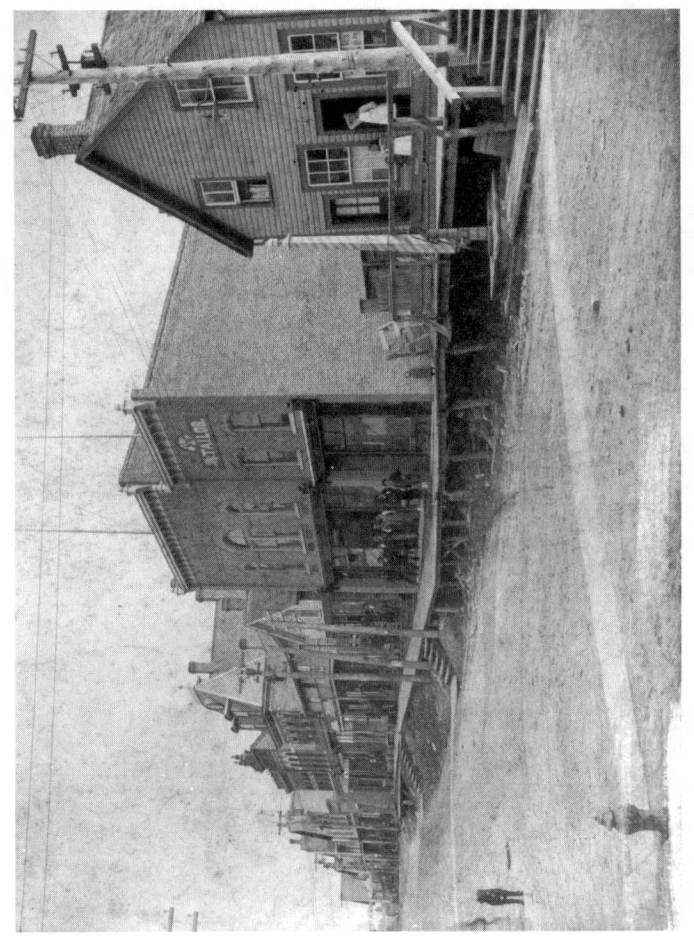

Customers and merchants scrutinize the photographer as he captures Manitoba Street, circa 1900. Even the dog eyeing the fire hydrant has paused for the occasion. The striped pole on the right signals the Joseph Caisse barbershop. Frizelda Caisse stands in the door, two daughters alongside. The child walking along the boardwalk profiled against the empty brick wall may be Rene Caisse. The house can still be found relocated behind the Owl Pen Book Shop.

A

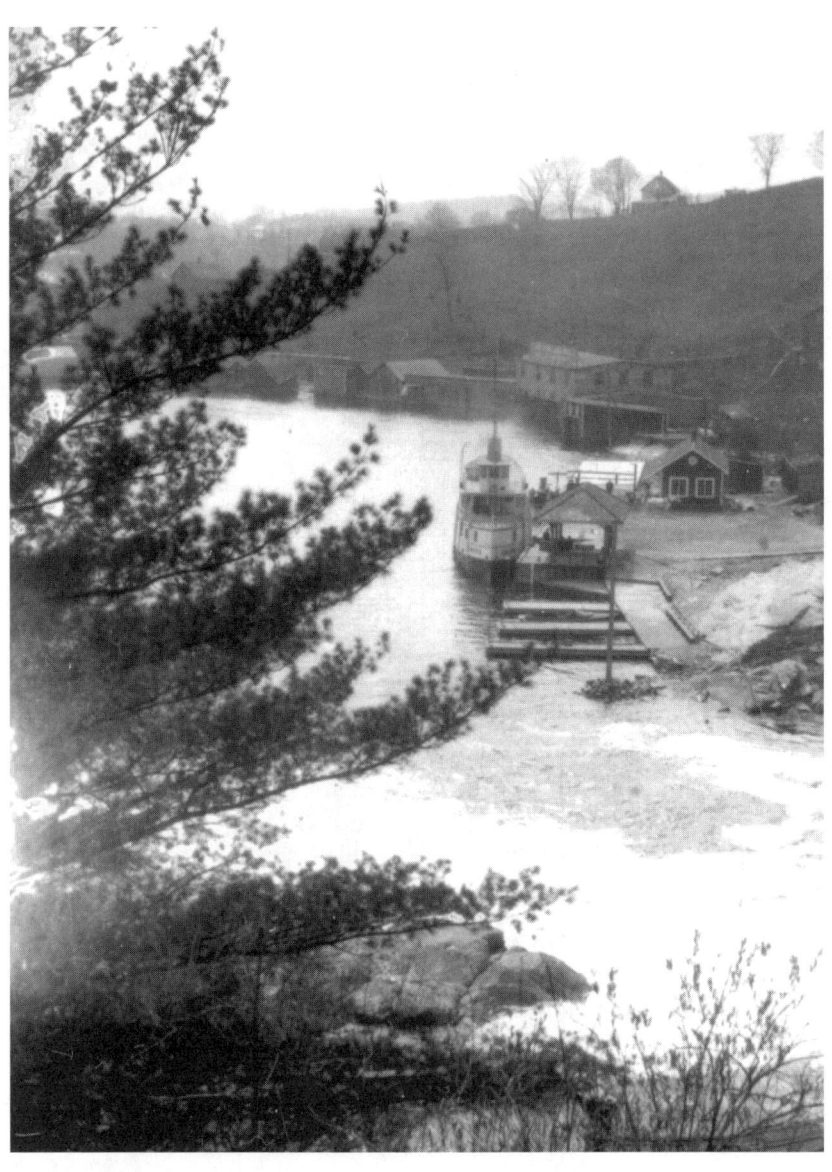

The steamer 'Island' May 14, 1914, the first year of the First World War was still bringing passengers to the dock below the original bridge at Bracebridge. It was on such a steamer as this that the Caisse's and other families arrived in Bracebridge.

B

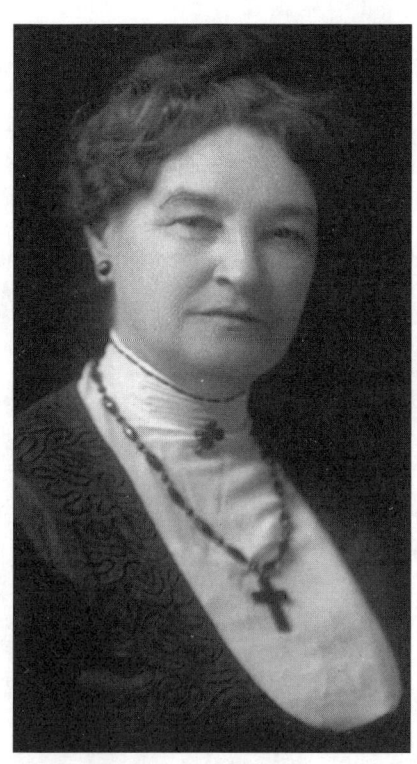

Frizelda Caisse who joked about preferring sons to daughters lived to be ninety, eighteen years added to her life after her daughter Rene treated her with the herbal remedy.

Joseph Caisse, well loved in Bracebridge, was greatly missed when he died in 1906.

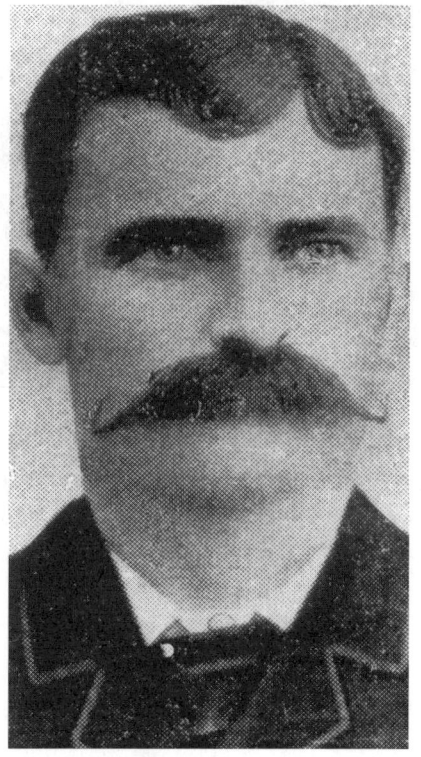

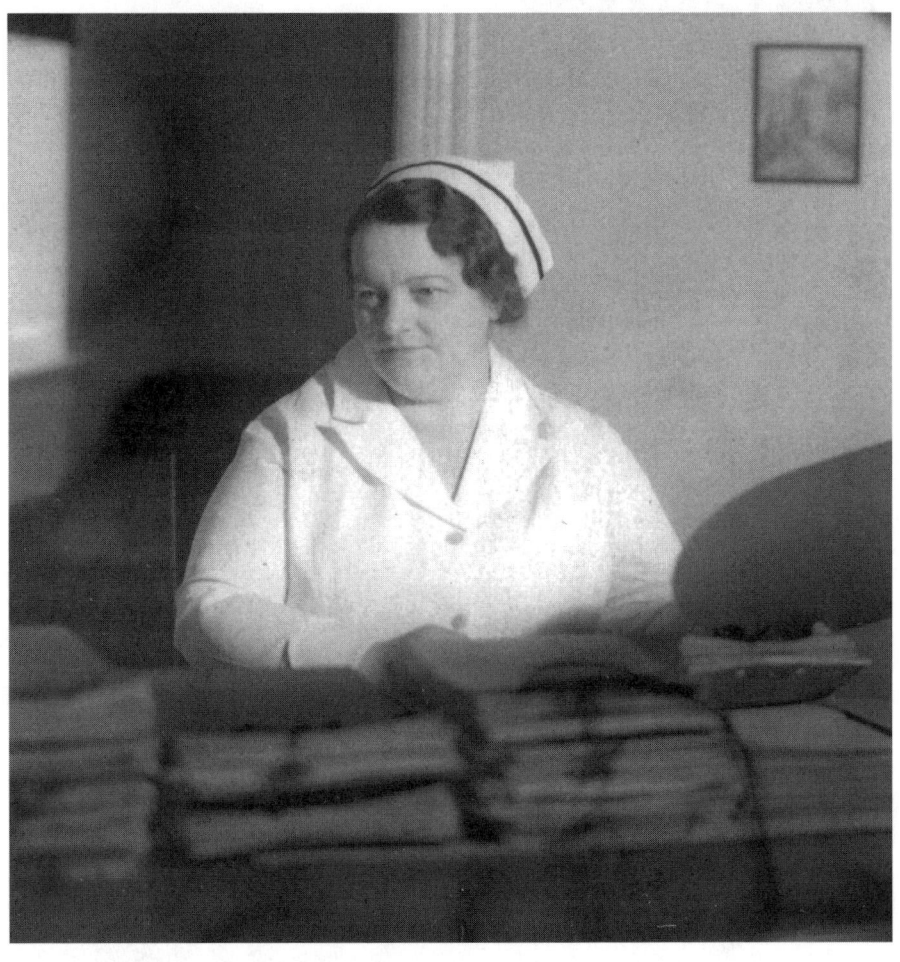

It was 1922 when Rene, then 34, head nurse at Sisters of Providence Hospital in Haileybury, met the Englishwoman who had been cured of breast cancer after taking a herbal remedy.

D

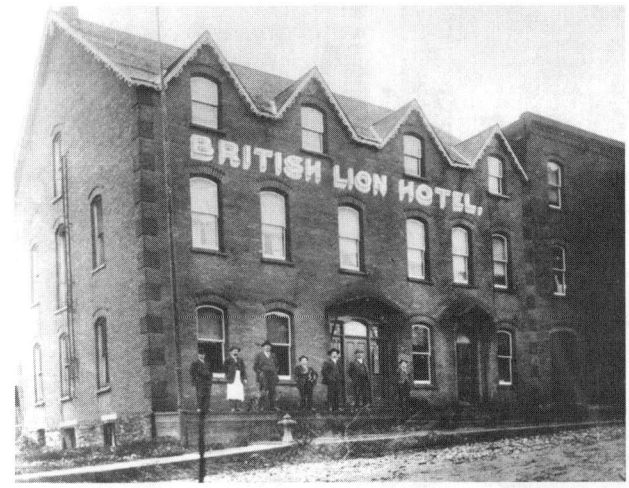

The old British Lion Hotel reclaimed for unpaid taxes. In 1943 at the urging of Dr. Bastedo, Mayor Richards and the Town Council rented it to Rene Caisse to use as a cancer clinic.

Today the Lee building commemorates with a plaque the drama that unfolded within, during the eight years Rene Caisse treated cancer sufferers here. Mayor Richards agreed with Dr. Bastedo. So did Town Council. They leased the hotel to Rene for $1.00/month.

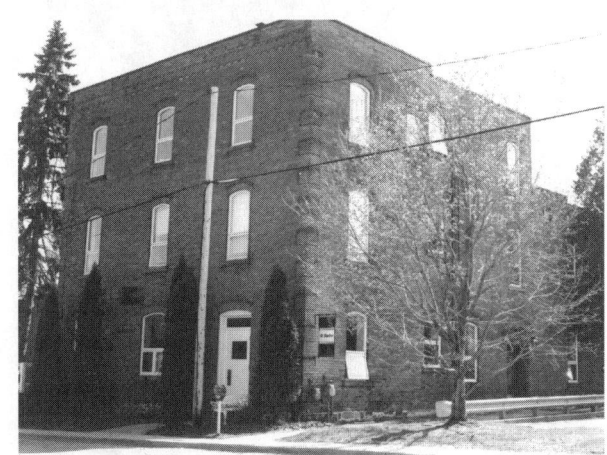

The plaque honoring the cancer clinic.

E

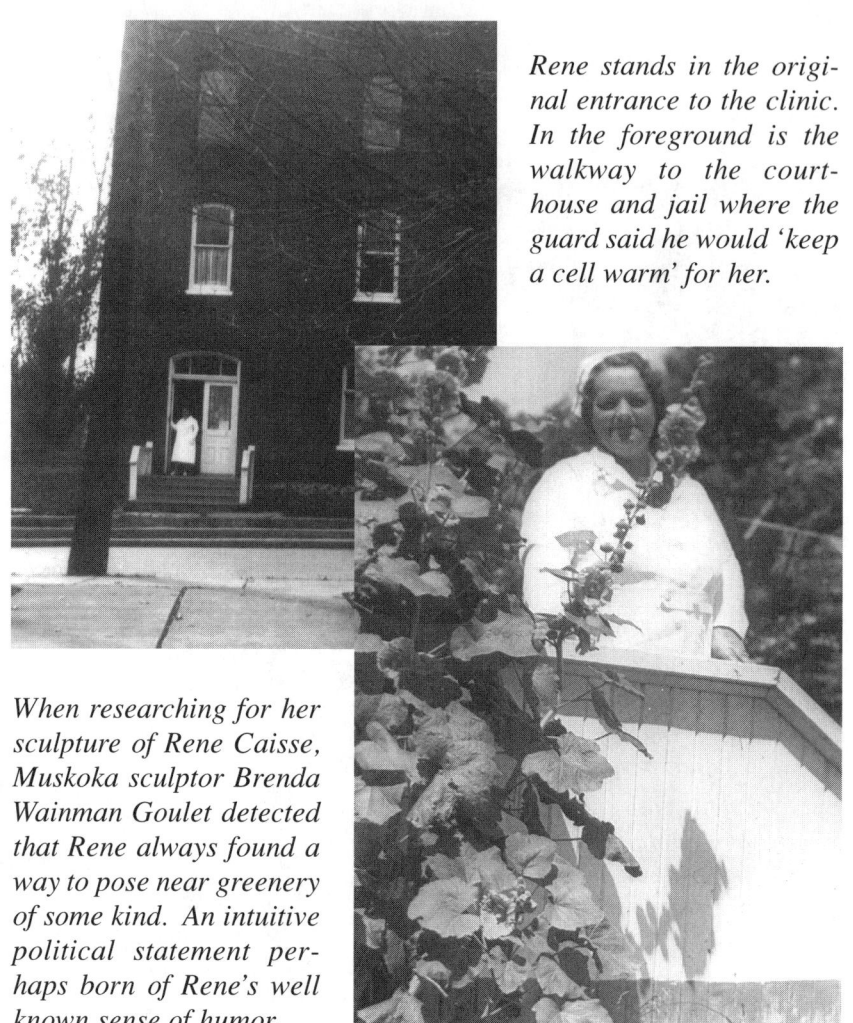

Rene stands in the original entrance to the clinic. In the foreground is the walkway to the courthouse and jail where the guard said he would 'keep a cell warm' for her.

When researching for her sculpture of Rene Caisse, Muskoka sculptor Brenda Wainman Goulet detected that Rene always found a way to pose near greenery of some kind. An intuitive political statement perhaps born of Rene's well known sense of humor.

You are cordially invited to attend a meeting in the High School Auditorium at Bracebridge, Ontario, on the evening of March 13th, 1937, at eight p.m.

The topic of the evening will be why "Essiac," the Rene M. Caisse treatment for cancer, should be given recognition by the medical world.

Doctors who have visited the Bracebridge clinic and investigated this work, will be there to tell the results they have seen. Any medical man who has suffering humanity at heart will be interested in this work.

The approaching election brought believers to Rene's aid, Premier Mitchell Hepburn among them.

F

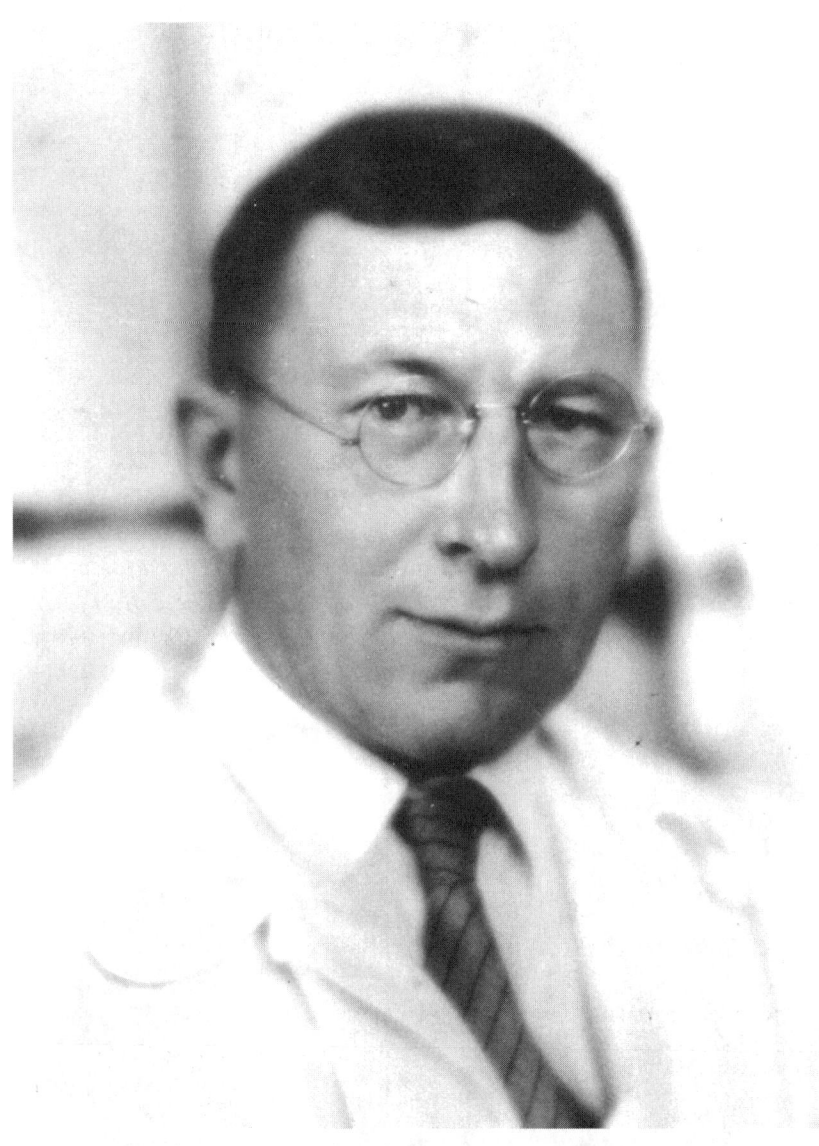

Dr. Banting offered to share his laboratory with Rene. Controversy still dogs Rene's 1936 decision to remain with her patients at her Bracebridge clinic instead. His professional respect for her lasted until his tragic death in 1942 while on his way to England with a discovery aimed at keeping wartime pilots awake.

G

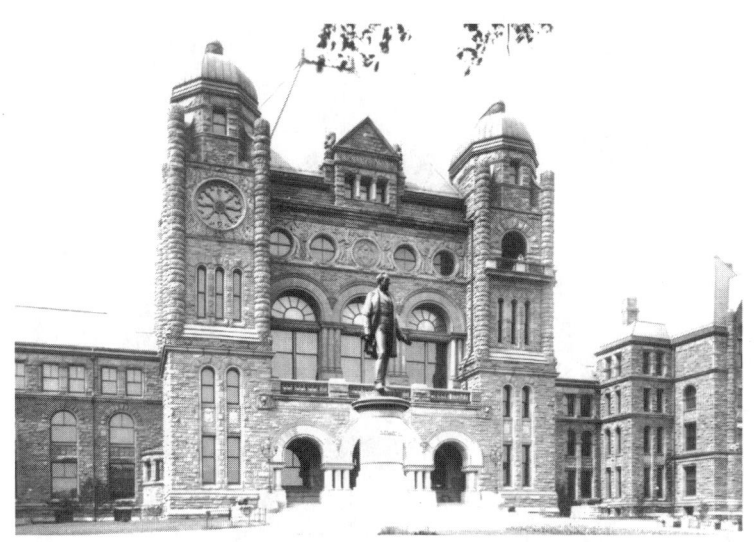

Queen's Park, where 55,000 signatures were not enough. Frank Kelly, MLA from Muskoka, introduced the Bill that would have given Rene freedom to tend to patients without fear of the law. The Bill in favor of Rene's treatment lost by 3 votes. That day the Kirby Bill was born.

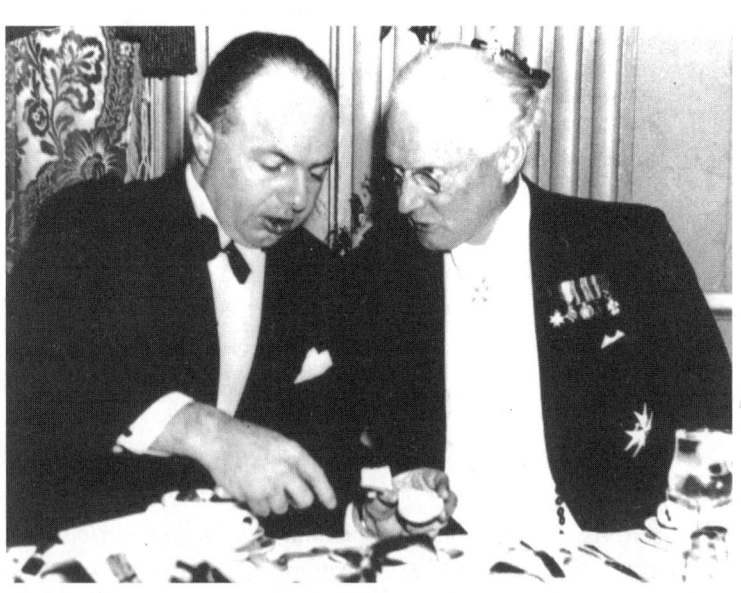

Premier Mitchell Hepburn of Ontario shown here to the left of Lt. Governor of Ontario, Dr. Herbert Bruce in the 1930's, understood what 37,000 signatures meant in an election year. But his respect for Rene Caisse was always genuine.

H

FROST & FROST
  Barristers
Solicitors, Notaries, Etc.

Leslie Miscampbell Frost, K.C.
Cecil Gray Frost

Telephone 41

Solicitors for
The Canadian Bank of
Commerce

Offices, Temple Building
LINDSAY, Ont.

June 4th.
1938

John Thornbury, Esq.,
HARTLEY, Ontario.

Dear Mr. Thornbury:

As arranged I saw Miss Caisse in Toronto on Monday and I thoroughly discussed her situation with her. In the meantime I have been receiving a number of newspapers from Muskoka District giving a further outline of the matter.

My strong recommendation to Miss Caisse was that she should sit tight and go ahead with her work. The undertaking which was given her in April was that she should not be interfered with. The Minister of Health, I understand, has renewed this promise and I do not think the medical people would agree to take any action which would stir up public opinion. I suggested to her that she should rely on these promises and go ahead with her work. She must remember that she has gathered great favour as far as public opinion is concerned and I think she would be making a great mistake to throw this all up at the present time.

I was very much impressed with her attitude and with her obvious desire to help people, and for one I want to say that I do not feel disposed to disregard any possible remedy for this disease. I, of course, do not know what line the Government is going to take nor what Commission they will appoint, but I certainly do know that the public expects any Commission to use a person of this sort with sympathy and consideration and not to close their eyes to any avenue of assistance to sufferers from this trouble.

I think Miss Caisse might well consult her solicitor relative to taking steps to protect her remedy by way of patent to prevent any disclosure adverse to herself.

This is a matter of some importance and I think she might be well advissd to consult a good patent solicitor in Toronto.

I intend to keep in touch with the whole situation and I wish you would keep me advised. Best regards.

Yours very truly,

LMF:J   Leslie M. Frost.

In 1938, long before he was Premier of the Province of Ontario, Leslie Frost encouraged Rene Caisse with this remarkable endorsement of her life and her work.

I

Below you will find a copy of the Minutes of a Council Meeting of the Town of Bracebridge, when, at Dr. A.F. Bastedo's request, the Bracebridge Council gave me the building I am occupying at the present time to be used as a Cancer Clinic.

The Regular Monthly Meeting of the Town Council was held in the Council Chamber on Tuesday April 9th. 1935.

Members all present except Councillors Gibson who was ill and Councillor Whaley.

Minutes of last regular Meeting were read and confirmed.

Hines-Hodgson, that By-law # 613 as now read a first second and third time be finally passed.
　　　　　　　Carried

Hines-Rawson, that By-Law # 614 as now read a first second and third time be finally passed.
　　　　　　　Carried

Hodgson-Rawson, that By-Law #615 as now read a first, second and third time be finally passed.
　　　　　　　Carried

Bastedo-Rawson, That this Council grant Miss Rene Caisse, the use of the Bracebridge Inn, at a nominal Rental, to be used by her as a Cancer Clinic, and that we give her a Lease accordingly.
　　　　　　　Carried

Hodgson-Hines that the Property Committee temporarily absorb the duties of the Road and Bridge Committee with Councillor Rawson as Chairman of the combined Committee.
　　　　　　　Carried

Hodgson-Rawson, that this Council do now adjourn until the next regular Meeting, or until called together by the Mayor.
　　　　　　　Carried.

Alex. C. Salmon　　　　　　　　Wilbert Richards
Town Clerk.　　　　　　　　　　Mayor.

In one of the most charming anecdotes in Canadian history, the Bracebridge Town Council led by Mayor Richards, at the urging of Dr. Bastedo, leased the British Lion Hotel to Rene M. Caisse for $1.00 a month so she could return to her home town and treat cancer sufferers surrounded by a supportive community. They furnished her clinic with odds and ends from their own homes.

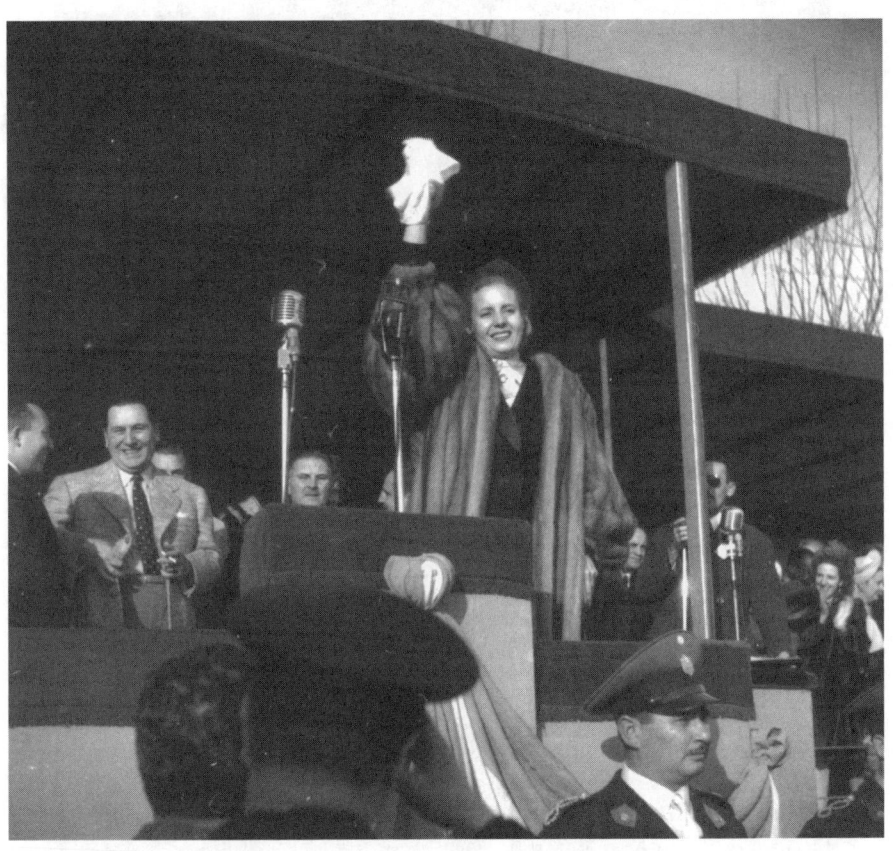

Stricken with cancer at 32, the living legend and folk hero to millions in Argentina and a media phenomenon worldwide, Evita (Eva Peron) waited for Rene in Duluth.

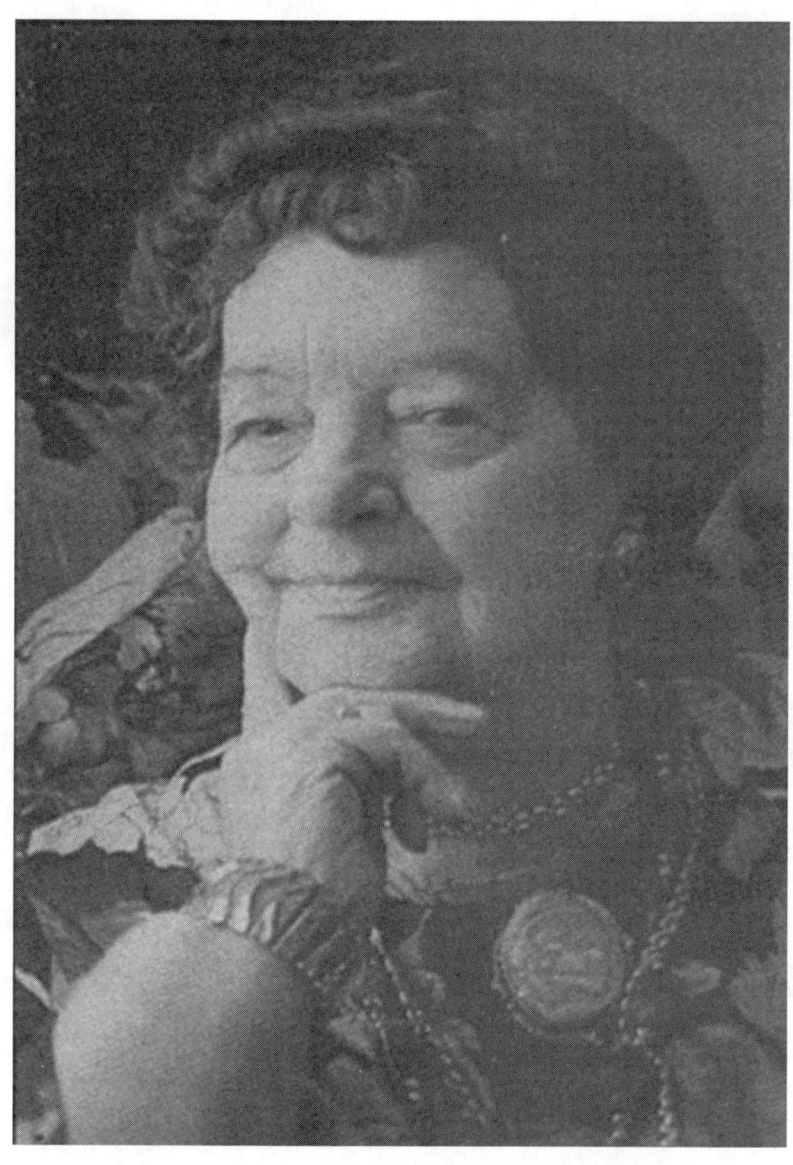

Rene at her last birthday. Former cancer sufferers, politicians, friends, and neighbors gathered in Bracebridge for her 90th birthday celebrations. A lifetime of affection was poured out for "Canada's Cancer Nurse."

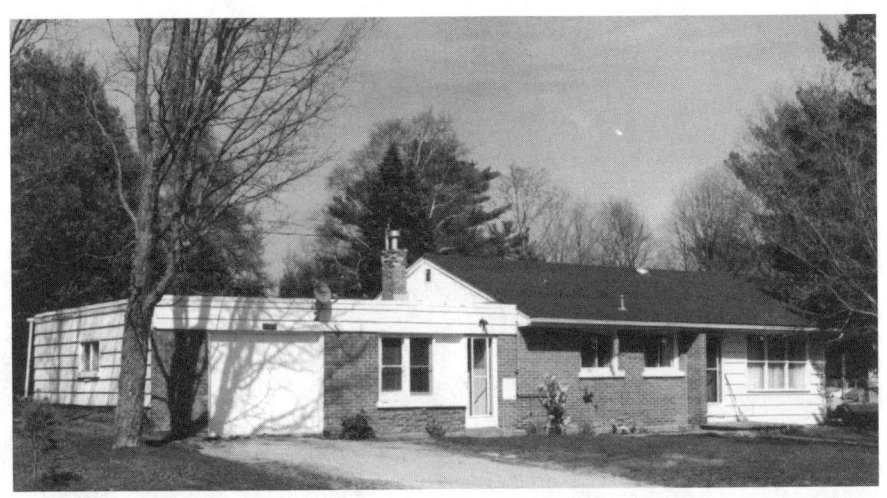

All her life Rene refused to take money for treating cancer sufferers. The remedy, she insisted, belonged to suffering humanity. In 1977, one year before she died, in her last modest home on Hiram Street in Bracebridge she signed over her formula to Resperin Corporation for $1.00.

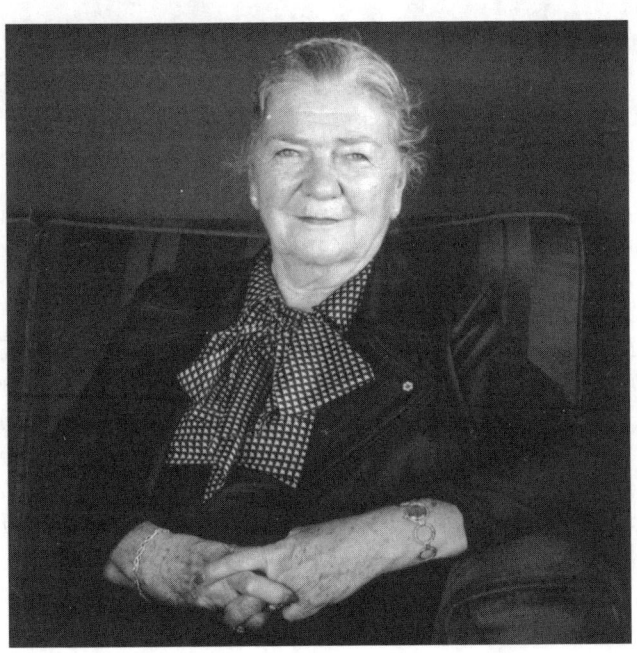

Lieutenant Governor of Ontario, Pauline McGibbon, came to witness and officiate at the signing.

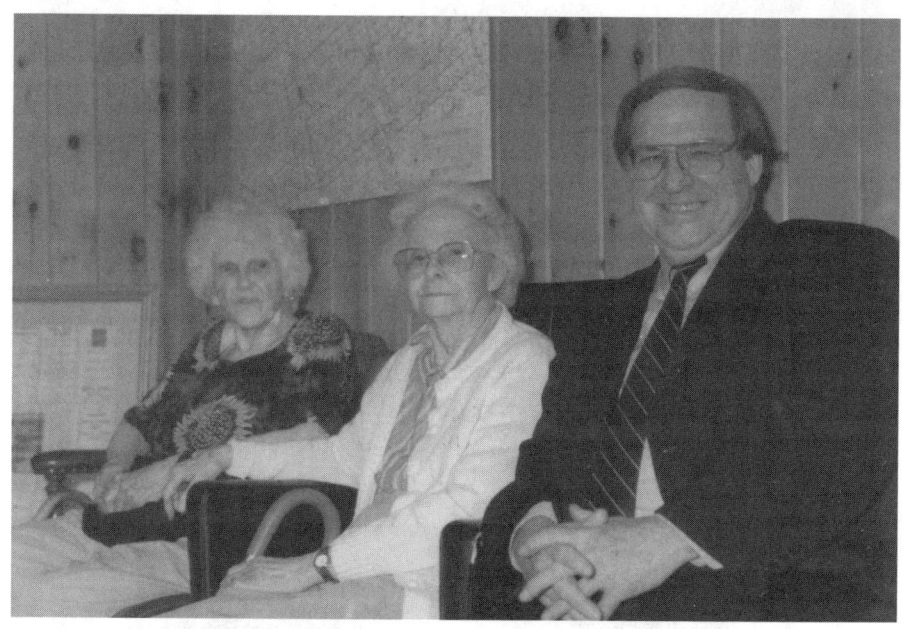

On June 21st, 2000, the Rene M. Caisse Commemorative Project was unveiled to Mayor Scott Northmore and the Bracebridge Town Council. Present was lifelong friend of Rene Caisse, Mary McPherson whose decades of hoping and waiting for clinical trials to be done on Essiac® were finally about to be fulfilled. Seated with her is T.P. Maloney, distributor of the authentic Rene M. Caisse Essiac® formula whose company Essiac® Canada International is funding the Rene M. Caisse Botanical Collection at the Canadian College of Naturopathic Medicine in Toronto, complete with 1) a Rene M. Caisse botanical garden 2) the establishment of an Academic Memorial Chair in the name of Rene M. Caisse 3) the Rene M. Caisse scholarship to a Bracebridge student who pursues a career in natural medicine.

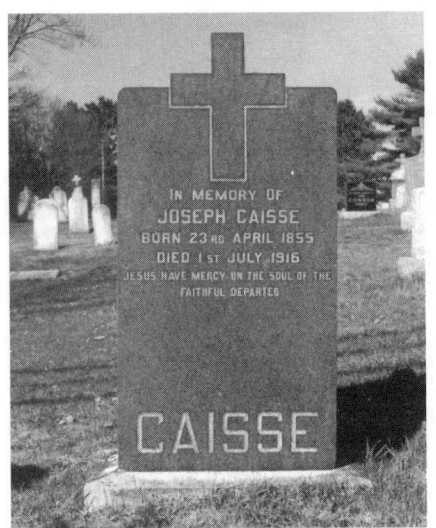
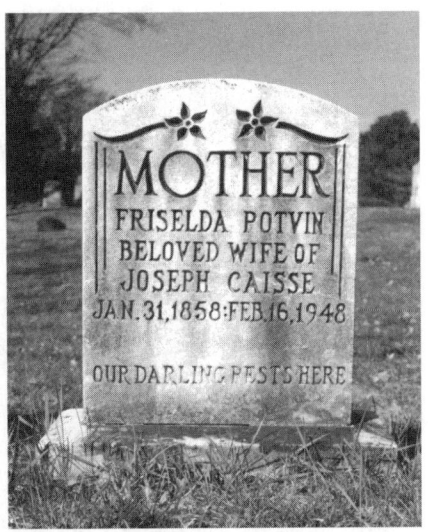
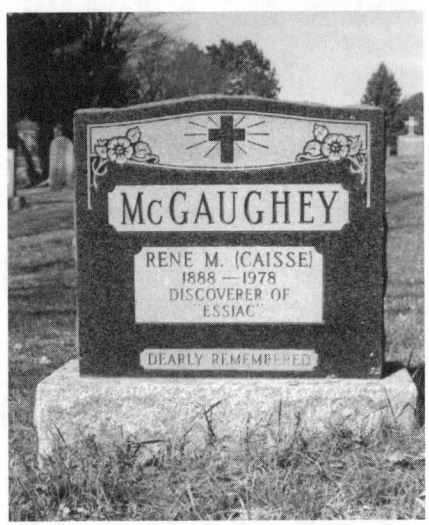

Their family crest was the dragon. Of her remedy Rene said, "It was so simple I didn't think anyone would believe it." Hundreds of thousands believe it today, many of them making the trek to Bracebridge to cross the famous bridge, visit the famous clinic and stand for a moment of gratitude at the roadside headstones of Rene and her parents Frizelda and Joseph Caisse.

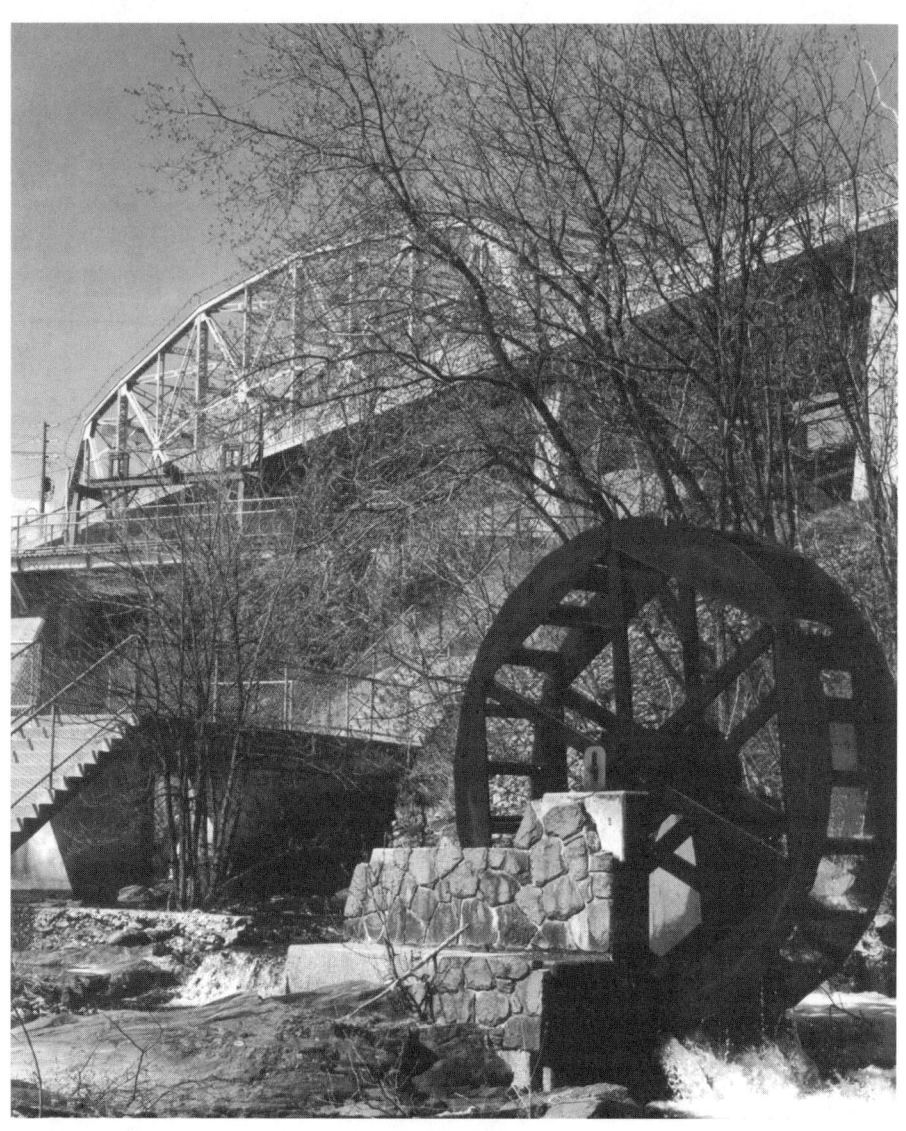

Most cancer sufferers arriving in Bracebridge knew only that to find the clinic they must 'Cross the bridge and turn left', passing overhead the famous waterwheel, a sign of hope since ancient times. Above, the famous bridge today.

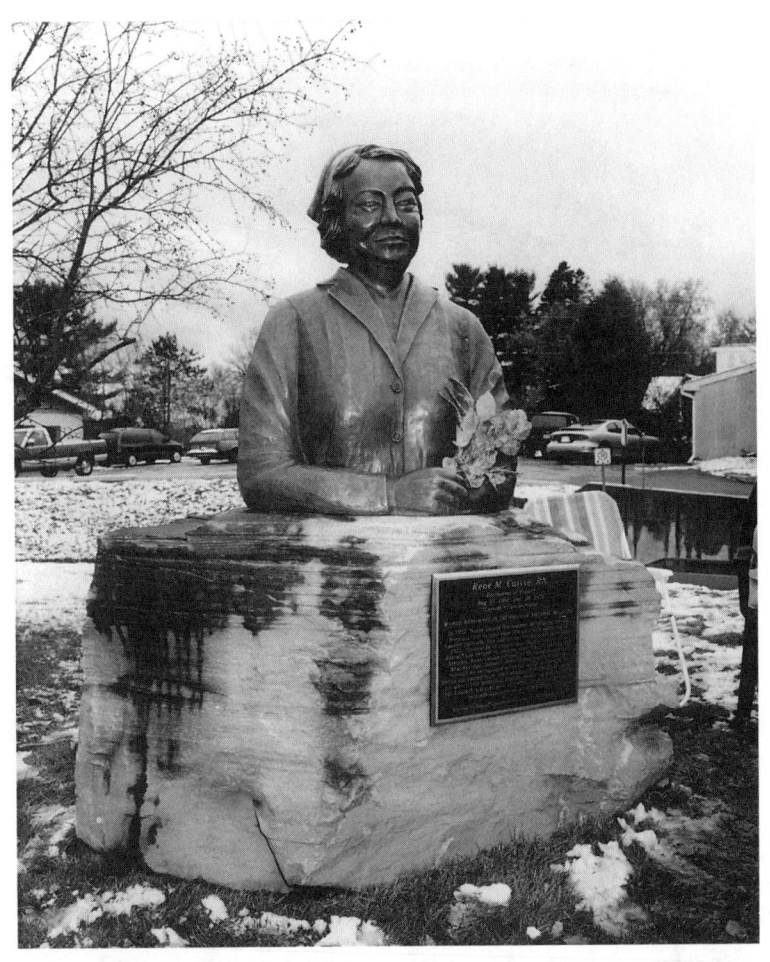

Bronze memorial on granite base with plaque at Totem Pole Park, Bracebridge, Ontario, officially unveiled by Mayor Scott Northmore November 15, 2000.

PART II

ACTS OF HOPE

"It will be in your power everyday to store up for yourselves treasures that will come back to you in consciousness of duty well done...things that having given away freely you yet possess."

John McCrae

CHAPTER ONE

THE POLITICS OF PERSISTENCE

It was inevitable that America would beckon. That was the American way, to seize upon opportunity. While the general public was being prepared by newspapers and politicians that 'War in Europe is inevitable', Gershwin was cautioning America to 'Let's Call The Whole Thing Off'. Europe between the wars was a landscape of endless breadlines, endless terrorism, endless coups. Meanwhile, there was no 'between the wars' for cancer. Year after year the lines were unending, families terrorized by the threatened loss of a loved one.

"The vast majority of Miss Caisse's patients," wrote the visiting Doctor Emma Carson, "were brought to her after surgery, radium, x-rays, emplastrums, etc. had failed to be helpful and the patients were pronounced incurable or hopeless cases."[1]

"In most cases," wrote Dr. Benjamin Leslie Guyatt, "distorted countenances became normal, and the pain reduced as treatment proceeded. The relief from pain is a notable feature, as pain in these cases is very difficult to control."[2]

The degree and severity of affliction was staggering. The response to Essiac even more so.

Dr. Guyatt recorded, "...open lesions of lip and breast responded to treatment, cancers of the cervix, rectum and bladder have been caused to disappear, and patients with cancer of the stomach diagnosed by reputable physicians and surgeons have returned to normal activity.

"In checking authentic cancer cases, it was found that hemorrhage was rapidly brought under control in many difficult cases."[3]

By 1937 the compilation of cures from Essiac was so overwhelming that a petition circulated by patients and doctors garnered 17,000 signatures.

Though unrecognized by the medical establishment, Rene Caisse had for solace the faces of her patients. As Gershwin's keyboard emphatically declared that year, "They Can't Take That Away From Me...'.

To the medical establishment of the United States, awash in research money, a cynical Canadian toiling in the cancer wards might have been haunted by the degree of difficulty in tending to the sick with an unauthorized treatment. But Rene Caisse was not a cynic. She was now face to face with a conflict that had always loomed as inescapable. Would the cure for cancer be given to the world through American patronage thereby becoming an American success story, or would Caisse be able to continue to maintain that the home of the cure was Canada, the northern forests and medicine men the true origin?

The steady stream of rumor about the miracle treatment Essiac, now fueled by 17,000 signatures, stirred the American medical field anew. In Chicago, Dr. Clifford Barbourka determined to bring

Rene Caisse to the windy city and effect a meeting with Dr. John Wolfer of the Alumni Association of the medical department at North Western University.

Not only was Chicago in the 30's a long way from Bracebridge, there remained deadlines to meet and stops to make along the way. The invitation to Chicago being accepted, Rene worked throughout the weekend treating her patients on Dominion Street, then come Wednesday she would be entering the King Edward Hotel just East of Young Street in downtown Toronto to attend to patients who had booked into rooms there. Then it was around the corner to Union Station and the train trip to Chicago.

At the border she presented the invitation and letter from Dr. Wolfer to customs before exposing the customs officers to the collection of natural botanicals in her luggage that might have had them mistake her for a prop assistant to Dorothy in the Wizard of Oz. The nurse from small town Ontario arrived in gangland Chicago where amidst the infamy of mafia power struggles and legendary police corruption, the true 'untouchables', the hopeless terminal patients remaining, as they always had been, proof that, even in inventive, fantastically creative and accomplished America there was no Yellow Brick Road back to health.

The files of many of the most hopeless cases had found a home in the office of Dr. John Wolfer. There Rene read the case histories of the patients she was asked to treat. All were classified 'hopeless'. Wolfer had expected her to turn down the opportunity. Instead, she sorted through them, then asked, "When would you like me to start, Doctor?"

Arrangements were made. She began treating the victims with Essiac under the observation of five doctors every Thursday. When asked why she accepted the challenge, she answered confidently, "I will show results that will surprise them even in the late stage of the disease. Enough to interest the most skeptical of them."

She did just that. The treatments lasted for a year and half as she traveled from Bracebridge to Toronto, then Chicago and back again over and over.

The results were convincing. Her Chicago colleagues and hosts through Dr. Barbourka, offered to open a Clinic for her at the Pasavant Institute in Chicago on the condition that she would remain in the United States.

She responded with a refusal. "I wanted my work recognized in Canada and didn't want to abandon my Bracebridge patients." [4]

There was another reason. That year Rene Caisse had become Mrs. Charles McGaughey. A barrister, McGaughey soon found himself the recipient of an offer presented on behalf of American businessmen through the American attorney Ralph Salt. It proposed to establish an Essiac Foundation with Rene Caisse at its head, investing $1 million to house and equip it, and to place Rene on an annual stipend of $50,000, this on top of royalties that would accrue from marketing the product. To sweeten the offer, they proposed to her an outright gift of $200,000. [5]

In 1937, dollar figures such as these would make any head spin. The Depression was still blowing dust into the naked empty bowl of the American farmer's heart. Starvation was a way of life around the world as it always had been, but the breadlines now extended around the globe right to front doors in Canada. In Saint Joseph's Church in Bracebridge, Rene's own mother Frizelda worked tirelessly along with many others to find ways to provide for families who could not provide for themselves.

Long ago Rene had determined that Essiac would not be exploited for financial gain, but might not another argue to Rene that it could be those very 'exploiters' who would create the means to have distribution of Essiac effected throughout the world? In that way it would at least reach some of the victims, albeit those with the ability to pay for the supplies. Another might say to Rene, come now, what do old promises and old standards mean after all? The concept of loyalty to ideals is changing, old values are shifting. Had not the King himself, last December 11, walked away from his throne and the responsibility and promises of centuries out of loyalty to the woman of his dreams, the twice divorced American, Wallis Warfield Simpson?

The nobility of romance was once again relegated by the newspapers to merely the state of being in love, that willing surrender to temporary dementia that is the common denominator of the spirit of adolescence worldwide, that spirit that so very often does not vacate the human heart when adolescence yields to the passing of time. What about the romance of healing? The romance of believing? Was life not a constant search for the proper suitor, be it in religion, science, medicine? Dreaming, hoping, was not only the domain of the young. There are so many ways to make love to a person, so many ways to make love to humanity. Yet, the thrill of infatuation, of lovers walking hand in hand, of dreamers seeking their dream in another's eyes spurs all onlookers to hope to pursue their own dream.

The Prince of Wales, with his renowned interest in the common man had long ago touched Rene's imagination. Among the myriad letters she had written and sent off in her pursuit of open-minded intellects who might turn their concerns for humanity to those suffering from history's most persistent plague, one had been addressed to the Prince of Wales. He had received it, his secretary presenting it on his behalf to the British Cancer Campaign. The Campaign in turn immediately afterward requested more information on Essiac.

She had addressed a personal plea to his father, George VI, as well, imagining that it might somehow end up in the lap of the stern but astute Queen Mary, who looking down at it over her neck high column of pearls, would have her intellect challenged by what was worded there. But now the King was dead, long live the King. The new man on the throne would not be King Edward, the prince of romance. It would be another.

Yes, the persuasive charms of Wallis Warfield Simpson could be felt even in conversations in the mid-Ontario town of Bracebridge. What did old values matter after all?

America may have been a champion of persistence. But Rene Caisse veritably refined it. As she would often say, "The love and respect of fellow man meant more than riches."

Her decision not to yield to the siren call of the American marketplace was an emotional, visceral one.

"...my forebears on both sides of the family had come to Canada from France in the 1700's and I had made up my mind long ago that Canada would get the credit for providing a cure for the world's most dreaded disease."

The Dominion Street Clinic of Bracebridge was not about to lose its nurse and its reason for being.

"Cross the bridge and turn left," even the well-renowned might utter at the sight of the bridge that announced they had reached the famous town.

Yet another doctor, Richard Leonardo of Rochester, New York, a renowned specialist who had authored books on cancer and studied related surgical procedures in Europe, stated bluntly that he believed she did not have any remedy.

Rene challenged him to stick around and watch. He did.

After visiting the sufferers in the clinic he did go so far as to state, "You're doing them good, but it's your personality and the hope you offer them."

Leonardo had put his finger precisely on one undeniable mystery of healing that had taken place around Rene Caisse since her early nursing days in Haileybury. His observations of her at work on sufferers is a veritable encyclopedia of nursing, epitomizing what was meant by Dr. Bernard Lown, Professor of Cardiology, Harvard University.

"Curing resides within the patient. The function of medicine is merely to activate this process and lend it support."[6]

But Leonardo reduced this to the cliche that the apparent cures were strictly psychological. Far from being offended, Rene then gave him a sampling of that personality trait that had endeared her to so many doctors before him. So confident was she of Essiac that she reacted to skepticism with wry amusement, never making the skeptic feel excluded.

She invited what she called, 'the big bluff fellow", to watch her in action in the treatment room. [7]

Inside Leonard saw cases far more advanced than those he had consulted with in the waiting room. He watched her labor with and comfort the victims until 7:30 that evening.

One of the cases he encountered would leave a lasting impression on him, be interpreted with very peculiar purpose by the medical establishment and simply stun the layman who heard of it. The name of the patient was Mrs. Annie Bonner, a resident of Logan Avenue in Toronto. In December, 1935, she had been rushed to St. Michael's Hospital here in Toronto by Dr. Stanley, who examined her.

Her words, "After having a section of the growth removed for examination, the doctor told my husband that it was definitely cancer. He told me also that it was inoperable as the growth had already sprung to my inner organs," evoked memories of the Englishwoman, Mrs. A., a prospector's campfire, and an Indian with a quiet voice.

Bonner suffered for ten days with radium needles and spent altogether nine weeks in the hospital.

"After four weeks' rest I started taking X-ray treatments. These were administered each day and sometimes twice a day for a year, except for occasional periods of rest..." that betrayed one of the most horrifying aspects of radiation treatment, "....when I was too badly burned to continue."

"By this time the X-ray treatments spread the growth up the right side of my body, to the right shoulder.

"At this time the doctor suggested removing the right arm from the shoulder.

"Needless to say I was feeling very ill and was unable to rise from my bed or even a chair without help."

At this time Mrs. Bonner's weight had reduced from 120 pounds to 90 pounds and she had suffered a complete loss of appetite.

A friend told her about the clinic and the nurse in Bracebridge. She refused to have her black and swollen arm—it was twice the normal size—amputated, so the doctors could do nothing for her.

She decided to make the trip to Bracebridge, so weak she had to lie down in the back of the car.

Cross the bridge and turn left...

Dr. Leonardo saw the arm. He said it was dead and would never move again.

"But after a few treatments I began to feel much better. The swelling gradually went down in the arm and my appetite improved. ...After about 60 treatments I underwent a series of X-ray examinations."

No sign of the growth appeared whatever.

Leonardo had been touched, moved, impressed and had talked to other doctors as well as patients.

To the nurse of Bracebridge he said, "Well, by God, you've got it! But the medical profession isn't going to let you do this to me. I've spent seven years in medical school and I've written books."

He would have to tear up his books, he said, throw out his surgical instruments if her treatment was ever accepted. [9]

Overcoming his original skepticism, he stated after visiting the Bracebridge clinic that her treatment would, "...change the whole theory of cancer treatment" and would eventually "...do away with the surgery, radium and x-ray treatments for cancer."[10]

He offered to equip a hospital for her in Rochester, New York. But again came the condition that she would have to live and work there.

Among the tidal wave of letters Rene managed to get out to the world, a veritable surf of them had for some time been washing up on the desk of the Premier of Ontario, Mitchell Hepburn. The 17,000 signatures on one 1937 petition, represented a block of voters no politician eyeing an upcoming election could sanely ignore. Hepburn was both sane and savvy. In July of that year he stood up from his desk to welcome into his office at Queen's Park, Toronto, the nurse from Bracebridge.

Here was a challenge worthy of the considerable tact Rene Caisse had previously bestowed on persons in the medical and scientific community. Hepburn was no less impressed than the thousands of patients and hundreds upon hundreds of doctors who had encountered her clear-eyed integrity and forthright frankness.

"I am in sympathy with Miss Caisse's work..." he said to the press. He could hardly have not said so. Cancer, in 1937, had a massive presence in the voting booths of the province. "...and will do all in my power to help her."

He added his commitment, if re-elected, to pass a bill in the legislature that would grant her a license to continue.

Very adroitly he spoke for cancer sufferers throughout his electorate, the thousands of patients restored to health by Essiac and the thousands who had been prevented from acquiring its benefits by the bureaucrats of the medical establishment.

With words well chosen to inflame the passion of the voters to Rene's cause and serve notice to the medical establishment that it had no power in the voting booth, Hepburn pronounced what would be certain to be tomorrow's banner headlines in the papers: "The onus is now on the medical profession. They must now either prove or disprove Miss Caisse's claims...," then he added those vote-netting words, "...and I don't think they can disprove them."

The colorful career and oft pugnacious roller-coaster personality of the rabid anti-unionist Hepburn was never more focused, nor more effective than in that choice of words, "I don't think they can disprove them."

Patients knew the claims could not be disproved. Rene knew. Her doctors knew. History before Hepburn's pronouncement, during that year and in all the years since has demonstrated precisely that the medical profession could not disprove Essiac's claims. The opposition that Rene Caisse knew was out there, the faceless, nameless monolith of the billion dollar cancer research industry might and did spend years avoiding the facts, distorting the statistics, detracting from the pubic stature of the nurse from Bracebridge, but not even in one instance did they ever disprove Rene Caisse's claims that patients treated with Essiac were remedied.

"Cross the bridge and turn left."

This time, August of 1937, the car rolling over the plank boards above the rushing river carried Dr. Emma Carson of Los Angeles who, on the strength of enthusiastic comments on the medical grapevine, had traveled to Ontario to see for herself.

Carson was coming to a Canada still dismissed by many in the words of Voltaire as "... a lot of useless ice."

Word of colorful characters and high drama was seeping its way out of Canada and into the world press.

On May 28, 1934, a 24 year old French Canadian mother of five children born individually in the short seven years since her marriage, gave birth to five all at once. The birth of the Dione Quintuplets of Corbeil, Ontario, thrilled and charmed the world. On March 27, 1935, the world famous author of the 39 Steps, John Buchan, was appointed as Canada's Governor General. December 23, 1936, another medical practitioner from the same region of Ontario was sewing his legend in Europe, Norman Bethune emerged in battle weary Madrid to tend to the wounded. As always, American medical practitioners speaking of Canada had the name of Frederick Banting on their lips.

When Emma Carson arrived at the Dominion Street Clinic, its mood and operating style had been well established.

"I have never before seen or been in any manner associated with such a remarkably cheerful and sympathetic clinic, regardless of size, location or number of persons; or attended a more peaceful, sympathetic clinic anywhere."[11]

What did she see upon her first meeting with the famous nurse of Bracebridge? She saw the same visage the patients saw, the same that had inspired hope in the most hopeless and drawn the trust of countless doctors. Below medium height in stature, Rene Caisse presented to the world a congenial, unassuming manner, pleasant of face, familiar in conversation, open to the world. But within the eyes resided proof of a guarded wise soul who was nobody's fool. That look was there for the perceptive to glimpse, that canvas of the intellect that unfolds within the eye to receive the impression of the brush strokes of fortune good or bad, critique it thoroughly, then allot it a value. Those eyes were the gateway to the world of healing of which Rene Caisse was the sole custodian. No doctor from any corner of the earth would ever see beyond what she held up to them unless invited by her to do so.

The meeting must have been a warm one. Carson had planned to stay 12 hours. She remained for 24 days and studied the results of 40 patients.

Carson noted that patients soon after their first treatment of Essiac were voluntarily abandoning narcotics and sedatives that had been prescribed by their physicians. She determined by her own professional criteria that Essiac was, without any shadow of a doubt, effective, calling Essiac the most humane, satisfactory and frequently successful remedy for annihilation of cancer that could be found at the time.

"It proved itself superior in every aspect to all else."

The strength of this endorsement and whatever additional satisfaction Rene may have felt as a result of it coming from a medical practitioner who like herself had had to make her way in a profession still regarded as a bastion of male supremacy, would be considerably shaken 6 years after it was written by the news that the profession had lost a fine intellect and a searching soul with the death of Dr. Emma Carson from a heart attack in California.

CHAPTER TWO

WHEN OWLS GET THE VOTE

Election night across the province of Ontario Essiac patients awaited the count while on Dominion Street in Bracebridge election handbills littered the waiting room of the cancer clinic. The handbills carried a picture of the Bracebridge nurse accompanying the statement that Premier Hepburn had given his positive assurance that, if elected, he would, in the next session, initiate legislation to allow the clinic to operate legally.

A promise is a promise is a promise unless it's voting season. As the song goes:

"... price of a stamp keeps getting higher.

"... cost of a lie can't stop a liar."[1]

Promises were made to be broken. Rules too, the rogues say, were made to be broken, unless they were rules about treating cancer. You could go to jail for that.

It had been fifteen years since the nurse on the handbill had looked down at an elderly patient in the Providence Hospital in

Haileybury and saw evidence of a revolution in cancer treatment.

The roaring Twenties were gone, the Depression had come and still lingered; through radio, workers the world over were learning they shared a common disadvantage; capitalists in their isolated bank tower enclaves learning they had survived the collapse of Wall Street with even more advantages, and the garrulous raging of a madman in Germany was causing the speakers on radios across the hemispheres to quiver and crackle with apprehension. Air ships the size of skyscrapers were gliding back and forth over the Atlantic, movie screens were talking now. Soon, they said, ticket buyers would be able to see the color of Gable's eyes. Memories of Valentino still filled housewives with yearning, ensuring the tango immortality, and husbands a patient stare. Few homes were without electricity. The frivolity of the Twenties had fled prohibition and taken shelter, it seemed, in politics. The steaming hiss of socialism had been punctured by Roosevelt causing the Bolshevik kettle to cool and everything old seemed a New Deal again.

Hepburn won the election. A surprise to no one who knew him, he kept his word.

Frank Kelly, Honorable Member of the legislature from the Bracebridge's riding of Muskoka, promised to introduce into the legislature a private bill to authorize Rene Caisse to treat cancer in Ontario. But before he could, it was 1938 and a Mrs. Gilrouth had fainted.

It was morning. The two Gilrouth sons worried about their mother's weak spell. They were preparing to drive her to the Bracebridge Clinic when she had fainted. Now they had second thoughts. Mrs. Gilrouth insisted, however, on going. The sons feared the worst - the doctor had warned them she might die suddenly.

Her doctor had already spoken to Rene on the phone, telling her that Mrs. Gilrouth could die anytime of an embolism, that she had an ulcer, which would not heal. He said he would appreciate it very much if Rene could treat her for whatever relief she could give her. He forwarded a written diagnosis of Gilrouth's case.

They arrived and managed to find a parking spot, although that day fifty patients were being treated, the streets crowded. Like all arrivals she had her diagnosis from her doctor on file in the clinic.

The sons helped her into the waiting room. From there she was able to walk into the treatment room unaided. Rene gave Gilrouth the first treatment. A minute passed, then two. Mrs. Gilrouth fell to the floor. She was dead. The two doctors on hand were helpless to do anything, while in spite of what had just happened, other patients who had come long distances insisted on receiving treatment. Rene was traumatized.

The news fed the headlines in all the papers.

"Woman Dies After Treatment At Caisse Cancer Clinic!..."

Knowing the CMA would be breathing hell fire, Rene struggled to remain calm, aware that all the successes of the past would mean nothing the next time the College of Physicians and Surgeons sent arresting officers if she did not prove she retained a firm hand on her whole Essiac proposition. Now was not the time to crumble.

Two pathologists sent by the CMA arrived to do an autopsy, Dr. Robinson, a distinguished pathologist, and Dr. Edgar Frankish, the medical Legal Expert from the Attorney General's Department.

They did not arrest Rene but they did convene an inquest which was comprised of a full court hearing with a jury of 12 men.

The Judge was to be Dr. Smirlie Lawson of the Attorney General's Department in Toronto, to be assisted by Dr. E.G.Ellis, the Coroner of Bracebridge.

In the upset and panic that filled every minute, every hour that ticked by, Rene could not find the diagnosis from Gilrouth's doctor.

"Somehow word got out that I could not find the diagnosis. It was mislaid."

The court convened. Rene rushed in just as it started. Fifty-eight patients she had treated the day Gilrouth died watched from the back of the room as the hearing got underway. Mr. Gilrouth and his two sons were also on hand, present for the purpose of testifying on behalf of the nurse.

Her lawyers knew that without the diagnosis their client was in for trouble. Before they had time to confer with her the crown Attorney asked if she had with her the written diagnosis.

"Yes," she said.

Her lawyers looked on helpless, not knowing that she had just found it. She drew it out and presented it to the Crown.

The pathologists Robinson and Frankish had, as part of their post mortem taken some of Mrs. Gilrouth's organs to Toronto for close study. They discovered clots in the pulmonary artery, one of them containing two fibrous tissue cells that indicated the clots were not recently formed. Being the direct cause of the pulmonary embolism, they could not be traced to the treatment by Nurse Caisse for there had not been anytime at all after the treatment for the fibrous tissue to form. The cause of death was agreed upon as 'pulmonary embolism'. Both pathologists stressed emphatically that the embolism would have happened anyway whether Mrs. Gilrouth had received the treatment or not.

"Death occurred as a result of an embolism in the pulmonary artery," the report read, "a condition brought about by a varicose condition. Pulmonary embolism had been evident for years." [2]

Rene Caisse was exonerated from all culpability.

Drained by the experience, older, sadder and wiser, she walked from the courtroom asking herself the question "Why did the CMA subject her to this?"

Was it revenge of some sort by any one of the countless attention hungry, unfulfilled, frustrated, bitter and malicious bureaucrats that gravitate to life and death issues out of a need for power? The government was poisoned with them. The Medical Association was infected by them. They were the disease of modern society.

Was it intended by powers that be to destroy Rene Caisse's reputation as a means of destroying Essiac? Was some adventurous manipulator calculating that with Caisse discredited it might be easier to access the secrets of Essiac, that dispirited and needing support she might finally yield up the formula she had kept so secret? Was it intended to destroy the confidence of her patients, to convince them to stay away from the Clinic, bring it to a halt and make her more vulnerable to commercial pressure? All of it was possible. But as Rene Caisse stepped onto Dominion Street, she knew it had all failed. More cars than ever jammed the street, more patients with hope emanating from their cancer-ridden bodies jammed the corridors. And as she entered the clinic for the first time after the hearing concluded, the touches, the muffled throats, the tearful eyes, the cries of 'welcome back', 'good for you', and 'well done' almost made up for the pain of the previous few days.

Frank Kelly's bill was presented on the floor of the House in March, 1938, accompanied by the signatures of 55,000 patients and doctors.

David Croll, Speaker of the House, had his work cut out for him when he arrived at the Parliament Buildings that day. The press crowded the corridors, as they had so often done, but there was a special flavor this day to their jibes and jests as he passed by. They had caught a glimpse of the diminutive nurse from Bracebridge entering the chambers and were relishing the high drama of seeing the House brought to a reckoning by the masses of supporters who came to be there to celebrate with her when the critical breakthrough was finally made. Three hundred patients, Rene's own pastor, the Mayors of Bracebridge and Huntsville and prominent citizens by the score accompanied her.

The Minister of Health, formerly Dr. Faulkner, the same Faulkner who had been instrumental in bridging the distance between Rene Caisse and Essiac and Dr. Frederick Banting, had been succeeded by the Honorable Harold J. Kirby. The power of 17,000 before an election had been proven. Alas the value of 55,000 votes long after an election had been won became all too quickly apparent.

Kirby announced that he was about to introduce legislation that would create a Cancer Commission for the Investigation of Cancer Remedies. That would be the only forum, he stated, in which the pros and cons of Essiac could be properly evaluated and only the Cancer Commission would be empowered to pass judgement on Rene Caisse's treatment. She could, however, continue her work until such time as the Cancer Commission would rule.

More bureaucracy. More overkill. If you wanted an initiative to be crushed, create a bureaucracy to evaluate it. It was too familiar. The nameless, faceless adversaries who would see her stopped, discredited, run out of Dodge, so to speak, now had a name, 'Cancer Commission'.

A cynic might wonder if membership on the Commission would require past experience at obstructing the work of this particular nurse.

Rene knew the scenario off by heart. She had been watching it take shape for a mile of Sundays. A conspiracy, secretive in its opposition then, subtle once, now not so subtle, was out in the open saying at last, "We're not a secret anymore."

Don Carrick, legal counsel for Rene Caisse, rose to speak for her.

"...patients and their relatives are reporting that doctors are refusing to give her diagnosis of cancer..." he began.

Muttering and rumblings and the clearing of throats turned the House into a Gilbert and Sullivan orchestration.

"and..." Carrick continued, using a word that had no doubt reached his ear from Rene's lips, "... that a cabal..."

The mandarins hooted their disapproval of this affront to their dignity.

"Untrue!"

"Shame!"

"... has been organized...

"Untrue!"

"... by the medical profession..."

"Untrue!"

"... against her."

"Shame!"

The uproar lathered and foamed across the deck of the table before Rene Caisse. She held fast. She had been on sinking ships before.

"My mother..." a voice cried out, piercing the uproar.

"My mother was a cancer patient...!" the voice continued.

An individual had stood up and was insisting on being heard.

"...yet three doctors refused to give her a written diagnosis for Miss Caisse, though they gave it to my mother verbally."

Thunderous applause broke from the gallery. There fifty patients were on their feet verifying the point.

Croll called for order. They refused to be quieted.

He called for the dignity of the House to be honored.

Still they applauded.

He threatened to clear the galleries, have them ejected from the proceedings. At that they quieted.

The Liberal Member from Parry Sound stood to back Frank Kelly's bill.

"I don't know whether it's a cure or not, but I certainly have seen people who have been helped by her..."

Fifteen years at the bedsides of cancer victims, fifteen years seeing them restored to health and the nurse facing down the male dominated medical profession was at last identified as "...her."

He said it again, albeit with apparently the best intentions in the world: "I've talked to practically every medical doctor in my legislature, and there isn't one who's against her."

Not even her adversaries had been so patronizing as to repeatedly call her a 'her'.

The 'her' from Bracebridge knew as she left the House what was coming. She was not wrong.

March 24, 1938, the bill proposed by Frank Kelly was rejected by the Private Bills Committee. It lost by three votes. As for the petition's request that Rene Caisse "be permitted to continue without fear of prosecution, her work with Essiac," allowing it, they said, would send the message out to the world that the House was endorsing Essiac and that Rene Caisse had the cure for cancer. [3]

Kirby, as the Minister of Health, followed through, establishing the Commission for the Investigation of Remedies for Cancer. It's formation was passed by the House in April. To become law June 1, 1938, and to be known as the Kirby Law.

Between the time of the founding of the Commission and it's formative statutes becoming law, Rene's attentions were diverted somewhat whimsically back to the northern terrain where the Englishwoman known as Mrs. A. had been led away from her campfire by an Ojibway Indian to be told the identity of cancer curing herbs growing wild in the highly mineralized soil of the Precambrian Shield. There, on April 22, 1938, the popular, much written about Indian called Grey Owl, died. His apparent devotion to creatures of the wild had seen him appointed by one former Premier as the unofficial keeper and guardian of beaver in his region, beaver cleverly trained to swim in and out of his house through specially cultivated passageways. Grey Owl had exploited to the absolute maximum the sentiment white politicians projected on behalf of their voting constituents to a dispossessed people who still were not allowed to enter white men's drinking establishments.

Yet an Ojibway, who had passed on his peoples' cure for the scourge of the ages, would continue to go unsung and the agent for his remedy's passage to the world at large would continue to be vilified.

When the Cancer Commission's mission statement became public it included the point that anyone treating cancer would be compelled to submit to the Commission the formula for the treatment and any details regarding the form or method of treatment. Members of the Commission, it continued, would be bound not to reveal any formulas so submitted but should they do so, no penalties would apply nor would libel or slander actions be permitted against them. Fines of $2,500 and a possible six months in jail would face anyone guilty of infractions against these rules.

Rene Caisse returned to Bracebridge. Crossed the bridge and turned. Entered and announced to the patients and staff that she was closing the clinic at the end of May.

In closing the clinic, she was being neither political nor treating the Commission with contempt. She was being true. Her patients, overcome with apprehension as they were, understood that very well. They had come to know her very well. Though they would not give up hope. They knew the nurse would not reopen the Clinic unless she was asked to do so by the Premier of Ontario.

Later, much later, Rene, like everyone else, would learn that Grey Owl wasn't even Indian. He was a hoodwinker by the name of Archie Belaney from England. Had a wife back there all that time. Hoodwinked her by disappearing. Swapped her and the sceptered isle for a log cabin in Northern Ontario and enough beavers to hoodwink every politician in the land, decades before anyone even thought of institutionalizing the art of hoodwinking as the art of 'being politically correct'.

The joke about Belaney would be: Q: Why did he call himself Grey Owl? A: Because owls give a hoot.

Now if only they could vote.

CHAPTER THREE

THE 'FOREVER' NURSE

It means my life! a patient wrote, pleading with the Minister of Health to reopen the clinic. The demands flooded in daily, bags of letters addressed to Premier Mitchell Hepburn. Hepburn proved once again that his interest in the treatment of the nurse of Bracebridge was amply accompanied by a sincere compassion for the cancer victims whose eloquent petitions flooded his desk.

He included Health Minister Kirby in his request for the reopening of the clinic and assured Rene that she would not be prosecuted under what was now called the Kirby Law.

In anticipation of the sitting of the Cancer Commission, a delegation arrived in Bracebridge early in 1939 to study the files of treated patients and to gather personal testimonies from patients themselves. The investigation of Caisse's cancer treatment was coordinated and led by Mr. Justice J.G. Gillanders.

By March the Royal York Hotel had been outfitted for the purpose of hosting the special hearing. Submitting findings to the Commission were R.C. Wallace, of Kingston, R.E. Valin, Ottawa; E.A. Collins, Copper Cliff; T.H. Callahan, Toronto; George S. Young, Toronto; and adding a touch of bleak irony to the appointment list, the name W.J. Deadman of Hamilton. [1]

Toronto, that year, that month, seemed more than ever before, a city surrendered to the mystique of what was once the Empire on which the sun never set, the world territory colonized by Britain when it was Lord of the Seas, regulated by laws forged in Britain, governed by bureaucracies designed in and perpetuated out of Britain. In anticipation of the arrival in May of the shy, reticent, reluctant Hanoverian, King George VI and his fashionable Scottish wife Queen Elizabeth, print and fabric shops were already at full tilt producing the flags and bunting that would festoon the streets upon their arrival. It was not merely royalty that was being welcomed, it was the reassurance that, what with the earthquake of the abdication of King Edward VIII and the tremors emanating daily from a helpless Europe, people would be gathering on street corners and straining their necks for a glimpse of stability, of continuity, of hope.

One incarnation after another of the 'Rebecca' whom Daphne Du Maurier had unveiled mere months ago could be expected to be seen clinging to lamp posts around the world pining for a glimpse of her Mandalay, yearning for Fate, into whose hands she had committed her heart, mind and dreams, to be kind.

As across Europe armies formed, evaporated, formed again, as borders changed and refugees crammed roadways throughout the terrified, tottering world, as Britain prepared alone for a High Noon stand off with Germany, a diminutive nurse from Bracebridge, no Rebecca of timid spirits here, led 387 people from Front Street, Toronto into the entrance of the Royal York Hotel for what was certain to be the pivotal showdown of her career between her unshakable certainty and the skepticism of the experts.

They had come by train, some of them, arriving at Union Station directly across the street, others by car, a seemingly endless caravan of automobiles, searching for parking spots while streetcars clanging to a stop discharged city dwellers Rene had treated around the corner at the King Edward over the years, and still others who had been rich enough or at least equipped with what was necessary to get them to the Bracebridge Clinic by train or car.

The excitement of being together for their great cause did not altogether free them from that frantic response to fear of war that was, in 1939, everywhere blurring the distinctions between cultures, languages, customs. When people are afraid, they indulge in trivia for the chimera of power it affords. The world was afraid, that was clear. Proof could be heard in the conversations in the lobby and corridors of the Royal York as they gathered. Surface chatter had a lot to do with movie stars and entertainment news as if the Twenties hadn't ended at all.

The perennial Canadian pass time of straining to find a significance for Canada in even the slightest headline was in full play. Wasn't it noticeable, one might wonder aloud, how Canada was finally beginning to filter ever so haltingly, awkwardly into the American psyche?

Well, yes, another might say, but America would never lose interest in itself. Was not Hollywood at that moment spinning out cinematic Civil War memoirs; Bette Davis had just earned an Oscar for her southern Jezebel even as Atlanta premiered Gone With the Wind in a whirlwind of nostalgia for a way of life that would never return.

Yes, but had not Bette Davis driven with James Stewart all the way to Calendar, Ontario, to glimpse the Dione Qintuplets? Then, too, there was Arlene Francis up around North Bay, but she was going to be in the movie about the Dione's so that was understandable.

Of course, there was that tornado in Kansas whipping Dorothy and Toto away from that fascist of a school teacher, into Oz where there was never a threat of war, only witches who melted in water, and a fantastical Emerald City. But, everyone knew that the Emerald City had been inspired by the towers and turrets of the green copper roofs of Ottawa's Parliament Hill, protected by comic guards costumed after the winter uniforms of Ottawa's theatrical Changing of the Guard because the director who had been born in Nova Scotia passed through Ottawa when he was a boy, and could never completely eradicate the thrill of seeing it all.

On and on the chatter would go there at the Royal York as it did everywhere people had good reason to gather. Keep the chatter, the trivia afloat at all costs, talk about anything and everything to distract from the fact that Franco was taking Madrid and about to reveal that the Spanish Civil War touted as a great romance between comrades was the most barbaric ever fought on European soil, anything to avoid acknowledging that one million Canadians were on relief, that Ottawa was giving away ten tons of butter to the poor.

Yes, tie every lamp post, every balcony, every railing with a union jack or a red, white and blue sash, turn every street corner into a theater of optimism. Commemorate in every way possible an Empire that had instilled its sense of order throughout the world, an order this very March in 1939 that stood threatened to the very base root of its British origins, thereby jeopardizing too Canada's very founding blueprint.

Once inside the Royal York, Rene produced a bit of theater of her own, having chartered one of the ballrooms in the great hotel to accommodate her 387 supporters.

A total of eighteen experimental remedies for cancer were on the agenda for the Commission to consider. It was only after 1243 pages of court minutes were recorded that Essiac was tabled for discussion. The announcement was made in the ballroom.

There, among the 387 cured patients were faces from the past that had come to mean so much to the history of the clinic and to Rene herself. There was the big handsome Ukrainian from Manitoba, Tony Bazuk, whose co-workers on the CNR in Capreol had raised money to send him to Bracebridge for treatment, his English much better now.

There too was Nellie McVittie, whose doctors had told her in 1936 that the only thing left that could treat her for her cancer was radium, who had come to Bracebridge and stayed for two months, getting immediate relief and never having had a recurrence.

There as well was May Henderson who remembered all too well the day she arrived on Dominion Street in Bracebridge, her color muddy yellow, her hair thin and lifeless, her blue eyes turned grey and stony, unable to stand up for any length of time.

So many from every walk of life, every denomination. Cancer was the great equalizer, one might have concluded, looking over those patients in the ballroom.

Not on hand but still living after all these years was Frizelda, her mother, who had been given only days to live and her aunt Mireza in Brockville who had turned her six months into decades and had never experienced a recurrence.

"For years," Rene recalled, "the ministers and priests offered special prayers in their churches that my treatment would be accepted by the medical world. These ministers and priests saw these patients come to the town very ill, and saw them improve, and recover from their illnesses, and as I had patients from all denominations they knew that my work was for the good of suffering humanity, and they prayed that God would smile upon it."

This was their moment, those 387 patients, to finally get a chance to pay Rene Caisse back for the treatment she gave them, the treatment for which she never accepted a penny of monetary reward.

"The look of gratitude I saw in the eyes...when relief of pain was accomplished and the hope and relief when they saw their malignancies reducing, was pay enough for my endeavor."

From 1922 to this day in 1939, her career, her life, had been devoted to relieving the suffering of cancer victims. In the world of radiation treatment the death rate was not decreasing but increasing alarmingly. Had the time finally come for revolution?

The first witness was called for questioning. The early statements were strong, direct, uncompromising. Dr. Benjamin Leslie Guyatt, curator of the University of Toronto anatomy department who had visited the clinic almost every month for a period of three years, and was a familiar face during 1937 when Dr. Leonardo and Dr. Emma Carson were coming and going, stated:

"I am satisfied that the patients I saw at Bracebridge were definitely receiving benefit."[2]

What had he seen? In 1937 he had written, "In most cases distorted countenances became normal, and the pain reduced as treatment proceeded. The relief from pain is a notable feature, as pain in these cases is difficult to control. On checking authentic cancer cases, it was found that hemorrhage was rapidly brought under control in many difficult cases; open lesions of lip and breast responded to treatment; cancers of the cervix, rectum and bladder have been caused to disappear, and patients with cancer of the stomach diagnosed by reputable physicians and surgeons have returned to normal activity."[3]

How many, Rene might have wondered, of those patients gathered in the ballroom were in fact actual confirmation of her theory on how Essiac worked. She had seen it function the same way so many times.

After a few treatments patients might notice an enlarging, a hardening of the tumor, then it would start to soften, pus and pulpy material would start to be flushed out of the system, and the tumor would simply be gone. Essiac, as she saw it, caused all the cancerous cells to relocate at the initial growth of the first malignant cells, there to succumb to the influence of the botanicals in Essiac, to shrink, be detached from their reluctant hosts' cells, and to be flushed out of the system.

Clara Thornbury, weighing 72 pounds with cancer of the stomach, had been carried into the clinic by her husband John. She now weighed 107 and was now once more sharing with John all the precious lifestyle responsibilities that a loving marriage imposes on its partners.

There too was Annie Bonner, who had so engaged the interest of Dr. Leonardo of Rochester. As a direct aftermath of radium treatment, her cancer had spread from uterus and bowel to her upper right arm and she had been admitted to St. Michael's Hospital in Toronto slated for amputation of the arm. She resisted and instead had gone to Bracebridge, where, after four months on Essiac, her arm which had been black and twice its weight, was back to its normal size, and she had returned from 90 pounds to 150 in body weight.

The case histories were not merely dramatic, they were headline making news. Hopeless case after hopeless case had been restored by Essiac. The Commission struggling for control of those headlines that would make or break their credibility, stopped calling on the ballroom of 387 witnesses after they had interrogated only 49.

Then the Commission fell back on the ultimate bureaucratic field play. Question the validity of the original diagnosis.

Rene watched without recourse as all the nameless, faceless medical establishment detractors and obstructionists who had thwarted her for years now made their presence felt through the Commission. A fool-proof format for bringing down what soon became evident as the Commission's pre-established finding was initiated.

Firstly, question the original diagnoses of the patients sent to the Bracebridge Clinic. Any observer might have concluded too soon that this tactic would only garner more support for the nurse from Bracebridge from among the doctors of the province, for questioning the initial diagnoses meant questioning the abilities of the doctors who made the diagnoses.

Dr. Guyatt, for example, calling upon his extensive experience and long career, stated before the Commission that he believed the cancer diagnoses were bona fide.

He would not state that he believed Essiac was the cure for cancer because, "A cure for cancer means 25 years," and it was still too early to know that many of the patients gathered in the ballroom would live 25 and thirty years and more after treatment.

Guyatt had never hesitated stating his faith in Essiac since 1937 when he said, "I do know that I have witnessed in this clinic a treatment which brings about restoration through destroying the tumor tissues and supplying that something which improves the mental outlook on life and facilitates re-establishment of physiological function."[4]

The risk of alienating the doctors was soon overcome by the second tactic, presenting affidavits sent to Dr. R. T. Noble, registrar of the College of Physicians and Surgeons, from some of the diagnosing doctors denying their own diagnosis. This Dr. Noble was the same registrar who had been the chief of operations to whom the arresting officer first sent to Peterborough so long ago had reported. The Cancer Commission had demanded pathological diagnoses and Dr. Noble stated, speaking of his own pathologists, that even pathologists can be wrong.

The Commission's heavy-handed way of dismissing diagnoses was so blatant, Rene's lawyer suggested that diagnostics, in general, should be the subject of an investigative commission. He also suggested that there had been direct pressure put on the doctors to renounce their initial diagnosis and evaluation of the treatment.

The target of the chair remained, as was expected, the secrecy involved regarding the botanicals of Essiac. They soon closed in on their target.

"What she is asking us to do is pass on the case histories she has given us, without the Board having any knowledge of what the substance contains, or the theory of this operation or administration." [5]

But 387 cured patients made minced meat out of this posing. Next, then, the target would have to be Rene Caisse herself.

Commissioner R.E. Valin launched the question that had so very often haunted Rene's work, and in so doing, opened up the personality scenario that implied there was a weakness to the whole treatment because of a hinted weakness in the position of the nurse toward the general public. It was the Commissioners who were the guardians of public health and the nurse who was suspect.

"If she has a cure, why would she deprive the whole population of that cure?"

The lawyer, Murphy, rose to give the one answer Rene Caisse had always given.

"They will treat guinea pigs and mice with it for a while, as they have in the past, and then they may say it's no good. And then there you are, at the end of the road, when apparently a great number of people are satisfied with the results they have obtained."[6]

One of those was Mr. Walter Hampson of Utterson, Ontario, originally brought to the attention of the Bracebridge nurse by Rene's first champion, Dr. Albert F. Bastedo, he who secured for her the use of the British Lions Hotel as a clinic.

He had squamous carcinoma of the lip and Dr. Bastedo had recommended urgent and immediate use of radium treatment. He was completely cured by Essiac, the only scar tissue left on him being that caused by the removal of a small nodule for analysis. He testified before the Commission on July 4th. His recovery was undeniable; still, the Commission would commit with Hampson one of the silliest pieces of judgement of the whole hearing.

Now, a sure sign that government appointees know they are beginning to look silly is when they come right out and say they are not being silly.

Absolute denial has ever meant affirmative confirmation when headlines are at stake.

Chairman Justice J.G. Gillanders said, "If I made a favorable comment and put my signature to it, and it was found to be pure water and the effects were purely mental, I would look pretty silly, would I not?"

At that moment to a ballroom full of patients whose only scars from cancer were radium burns, the proposition must have seemed pretty silly indeed.

He added, "On the other hand, if it contained something harmful, I would still feel pretty silly."

Silliness was fast becoming as great an epidemic as cancer. It was affecting everyone. What could one expect after all in a time when the Prime Minister of Canada, Mackenzie King, whom history would reveal communicated with his dead mother by talking to his dog, had sent to Prime Minister Neville Chamberlain, upon Chamberlain's return from Munich waving the infamous 'Peace In Our Time' scrap of paper with Hitler's signature on it, "Your achievements in the past month alone will assure you an abiding and illustrious place among the great conciliators."

The nurse from Bracebridge could see clearly what the outcome would be when Commissioner Valin stated, "The treatment of cancer is the practice of medicine. She really is privileged. I do not think there is anywhere else in any other province in this country where she would be allowed to have a clinic and treat patients."[7]

Silliness, as a sign of the times, had begun to replace sanity: a Quebec tavern owner had to go all the way to the Supreme Court over the right to sell beer to a black man.

Silliness, as a sign of the times, had begun to replace charity. At the same time as the country was turning itself inside out to wave Union Jacks at the King and Queen of England, 907 Jewish refugees from Nazi Germany were being refused entry into Canada.

Then Valin pronounced the death knell on Rene's freedom to treat patients.

"We want to continue this investigation with some control in the future of cases which she will treat - that they would be seen by some member or representative of this Commission, and a complete diagnosis and examination done, and then follow the cases and after a certain time make a report. We feel we should like to pursue our observations further, and that is the reason why we want the formula."[8]

In fact, Valin had just stated what had been the bottom line all along: "We want the formula."

Would she yield? No.

"It is the opinion that the evidence adduced does not justify any favorable conclusion as to the merit of Essiac as a remedy for cancer.

"If, however, Miss Caisse is desirous of having the treatment further investigated, and wishes to submit further evidence and is prepared to furnish the formula for Essiac, together with samples thereof, the Commission would be glad to make an investigation in such manner as is deemed desirable and warranted."

To such a body as this Rene Caisse was expected to '...furnish the formula for Essiac...?"

Would she yield? Not likely.

The third tactic employed by the Commission was to accredit cures to anything other than Essiac. They had attributed the saving of Annie Bonner's arm to radiation even though the diagnosis given Rene when she met Mrs. Bonner read: "This is to certify that Mrs. Annie Bonner, 260 Logan Ave., Toronto, had been receiving treatment at St. Michael's hospital for cancer of the cervix. She has developed metastasis in the upper right arm." It was signed by Dr. J.C. Theobald, M.D. Bonner was told amputation of the arm was her only hope. One Dr. Connell had refused Bonner's case stating that the case was too far advanced for his treatment. She went to Bracebridge and that day at the Commission had an arm healthy enough to swing at any of the sitting specialists, which she might just have done, so angered was she by their false presentation.

"....thanks to Essiac my arm is normal," she would write to Rene."...I thank God for having spared me and sincerely hope that you may be able to carry out this work and eventually be able to make your treatments available to all cancer sufferers."

The Commission, incredibly, attributed the cure of Mr. Hampson to surgery and thereby lost whatever credibility it had managed to sustain throughout the Hearing to date.

The Commission stated that of the witnesses heard, there were 3 wrong diagnoses, 10 that were doubtful, 4 were termed 'not positive'

They did condescend to admit there was one recovery with Essiac and two improvements - the diagnosis had been made by biopsy. The same for diagnosis by X-ray.

Rene's single consolation was that Essiac, of the 18 remedies examined by the Commission, was the only one to be granted the recognition of having wrought any cure. [9]

To everyone's delight, the case singled out for credibility was that of Tony Bazuk, the big Ukrainian CNR rail man from Capreol whose struggle with cancer had been converted to a struggle with the English language. He was winning that battle too. His big smile and sympathetic grateful eyes would linger as one of the sole comforts in the wake of the Royal York Commission hearing.

By the time the Commission's findings were officially published the 'phony war' that haunted Britain all summer had finally ended. The world was at war. Rene Caisse was back in Bracebridge, the 'phony peace' with the Cancer Commission looming as just as bitter a farce.

From the railing of the bridge that marked the entrance to the town of hope, the narrow frothing river might drown out the pain of the memory of all those quiet, bleak faces in the ballroom of the Royal York as the hearing ended.

Solitude was the necessary requisite of innovators. It was 1939 after all, the age of dictators. Who more than Rene knew that the prevailing spirit of modern medicine had been that of striving for dominance and domination, rather than direction.

She was all too well aware that, "if anyone steps out of line and does his or her own thinking and accomplishes anything out of the ordinary with medicine and methods generally unknown, the dictators ostracize and condemn them without a fair investigation. No matter how much greater his or her accomplishment is than those of the dictators, they are 'quackific' and not 'scientific'. He or she is a quack or an exploiter."

Case in point: the Commission, after Dr. Connell had refused Annie Bonner whom Rene was able to cure, not only ignored Essiac, but recommended Dr. Connell for a grant of $25,000.

But the truth is,"...the lone thinker...has become so absorbed and interested in the results obtained that he or she, suddenly awakens to the fact that they have been exploited of everything they possessed."

Here in Bracebridge, Rene had sustained the courage to withstand the pressures of the world beyond, the lures, the promises, the threats. Here, among friends and supporters, she was strong. Did not scripture itself demonstrate that Christ removed himself from the company of doubters in order to produce miracles? Here in Bracebridge she was able to re-affirm her perennial determination.

Would she yield? No.

"Until the medical profession will admit from the cases I have treated that my treatment has merit, I will not give up the formula. When they do that, I will be willing to give my treatment to the world."

The litany of misrepresentations resulting from the Commission hearing prompted Rene to call it 'one of the greatest farces ever perpetrated in the history of man.' The list of deliberate slights seemed endless: over 387 witnesses had come to be heard but only 49 were called, then the Commission reported that Rene had only brought 49 cases to be heard. The x-ray reports were not accepted as diagnosis; 49 doctors, according to the Commission, had initially made wrong diagnosis.

When, after the Commission hearing had come and gone, she asked for a new hearing by the Registrar of the College of Physicians and Surgeons, they said if she treated any more patients they would take her to court.

Would she yield? No.

THE 'FOREVER' NURSE

Rene Caisse was a nurse forever, as they say of priests, 'a priest forever in the order of Melchisedech'. She was a nurse forever in the order of, perhaps, Veronica, a 'true icon' of the suffering of her patients.

And that she would remain for as long as the grass grows and the river flows under this famous bridge that had given so much hope to the hopeless.

PART III

A SINGULAR ACT OF CHARITY

"The girls who make music will not hear it said of me that I hide among the rocks. Is it not true that thrice I fell, and thrice I was picked up, and that, unconscious, they tied me with cords on the back of a camel? And, because of that, Defeat was no dishonor."
Anonymous Touareg Warrior, May, 1802.

CHAPTER ONE

THE GREEN-EYED MONSTER

"Power and the law are not synonymous. In fact they are frequently in opposition and irreconcilable"
- *Cicero*

Jealousy. It disfigured man. It had disfigured the whole cancer industry. "The jealousies and antagonisms of the cancer research workers in this country have delayed the cure for cancer, many, many years."

The charge made by Dr. I. MacDonald resonated credibly with Rene Caisse. The words of MacDonald, the Director of the Biochemical Research Foundation of the Frankwood Institute of Philadelphia, were not a revelation to anyone in the research field. Wherever doctors and researchers, profs and students were competing for credits and honors, the workplace could be guaranteed to be a minefield of acrimony, mistrust, accusation and counter accusation. It had ever been so. The poison fomented in grad school invariably congealed and lay like an old scum on the surface of this medical endeavor or that scientific adventure. Wherever the dictatorship of the prof/student relationship was allowed to linger in the research community, the contaminate of jealousy crippled innovators and turned pioneers into overprotective, defensive bureaucrats, legislating from the much guarded security of their own desk petty restrictive rules and regulations for their unfortunate subordinates to endure. Many an aspiring medical student or scientific researcher has seen his/her career sink out of sight below the surface of the ocean of educational peer publications controlled by the contemporary faculty tyrants.

"A number of years ago," wrote Dr. MacDonald, "I thought it would be a grand idea to correlate all the research on cancer then in existence to prevent undue duplication, and that each would get the advantage of the others' work.

"But I found that university men who make up the workers were very jealous of their plans and results.

"They considered their advancement within the University to be dependent upon their reputation as gained by publication."

Could an issue so vital as a cancer cure be denied the suffering public because of inter-departmental squabbling in this college or that university. Alas, absolutely. It is a world of calculated favors, limitless exploitation of subordinates, seething unbridled arrogance, favors called in.

"It seems almost unbelievable that the fullest advantages of research in so vital a field of medical science as cancer treatment, should be denied to the public for any cause, much less from professional jealousy."

In the months following the Cancer Commission's published report, written diagnoses from doctors for patients seeking Rene's treatment were almost impossible to obtain. The isolation of the nurse from Bracebridge was becoming more and more intense with every passing day.

The Kirby Bill was never enacted against her, yet, even though no charges were laid, she lived in fear of charges and imprisonment.

The romance of far off exotic medical opportunities must have appealed to her at that time, if only in escape fantasies. But the reality of high adventures came home all to clearly with the news that on November 12, 1939, Dr. Norman Bethune had died in northern China. His politics aside, Bethune had gone it alone, never shying away from a frontier.

In face of the fact that there was now a seven year penitentiary sentence facing anyone who gave out anything to help a cancer patient, Rene Caisse re-evaluated her profession and her life in it.

"The 'Cancer Control Society' in my opinion, is the richest and most powerful organization in the world. More powerful than any government, and are answerable to no law of any country. They have their own Police, they set up their own courts of law to deal with any one who is daring enough to have the courage of his convictions, and tries to evolve anything that is beneficial in the treatment of cancer, which is in my opinion their monopoly.

"I believe that they also control the Press, at any rate it is not healthy for any paper to print anything favorable about a cure for cancer.

"You know that when a cure for cancer is accepted, it will revolutionize the present day method of treatment, and you may be sure the Cancer Control Commission will never allow that to happen. They would lose control of all the moneys given them so freely for Cancer Research.

"This in my opinion they will never allow to happen, even though they have had so much money for research, they have not in fifty years been able to offer the world even a hope of a real cure for this most dreaded of diseases.

"The public are only told what the Cancer Society wants them to be told, and the gullible public accept anything they are told."[1]

Mankind the world over was in torment. France had fallen. Nazis and Fascists seemed unstoppable. In the cancer wars the thing devouring Europe resonated with appalling familiarity — all through '39, '40 and '41, as Churchill testified, the Allies never won a battle, the dictators never lost. The turning point in the battle with the Axis powers was still months away. But there would be no El Alemein for the solitary foe of cancer just up hill to the left of the bridge in the town that had done so much to support her.

How much better off might she have been had she simply followed the lines of least resistance, accepted the offer of the most respected mind in medicine, Dr. Frederick Banting, and put her research under the protection of his laboratory.

Should she have yielded then?

The riddle must have reached especial poignancy in 1941 when Rene heard that on Feb. 23, the plane carrying Banting to England with his newly discovered device for keeping pilots from blacking out, had crashed near Musgrave Harbour, Newfoundland. The report that emerged later of Banting spending his last hours, knowing he was dying, dictating notes non stop for hours to no one in particular, touched deeply those thousands in the medical profession whose lives involved an endless filing of uncountable mental notes, never knowing if they would ever be retrieved, read or understood. To Rene Caisse, whose home was reputed to be bulging with notes and files and forms, the anecdote of Banting, mentally organizing his legacy of notes in the snow outside the plane, must have had special poignancy. The war was devouring the planet and the best minds with it.

In 'a state bordering on nervous exhaustion', Rene closed the doors of the clinic in 1942. Fear of imprisonment was just half of the reason. Fatigue and depression were mated to it. Was she yielding to those faceless, nameless forces out there? Only time could tell.

The road out of Bracebridge led northward, away from Toronto and the seat of the Cancer Commission. With her husband, Charles McGaughey, she re-entered that world where the air tasted always new, the snow remained white long after it fell, and North Bay, the city of their destination, was so uncluttered of industrial sound that one could hear the neighbors talking a mile away.

The lake on which the city stood, the Nipissing, took its name from the Nebocerini who in 1649, in an effort to escape the clutches of the nameless, faceless Iroquois, those marauders who would study their victims from the shelter of the tree line then come forward and rob them of everything they had, including their lives, had put Lake Superior between themselves and their heritage. But for Rene, North Bay was far enough. The nameless, faceless bureaucrats inside the establishment tree line might take her practice away from her but they would never take her heritage. She would remain here in the middle of the province as middle age came and went. Mid-Ontario meant family, home and personal heartland. Here she would, at last, and for the first time, lead a normal life.

Here, defeat held no dishonor.

She had fought the odds since 1922, that Essiac would be accepted. Even men who had beaten the odds had no guarantee of 'happy ever after'. Murder in Nassau had claimed the man who had always succeeded in doing things his way when so few others could. Harry Oakes had been found dead in bed of blows from a blunt instrument, the title of 'Sir' accorded him for a life time of achievement by the British Government adding not one iota of security to him in his search for a normal life.

Rene remained on the banks of the Nipissing throughout the

War, during the first four years of which America lost 284,000 men in action.

In the same four years, Canada, with a population of a mere 11,300,000 managed to send 730,625 men and women to war. In the same four years America lost 672,000 to cancer [2].

The physician poet, John McCrae, whose 'Flanders Fields' had forever trapped in poetic amber the loneliness of the front line warrior, had also provided for the medical pioneer phrases emblematic of the martyrdom of the unsung researcher.

"It will be in your power everyday to store up for yourselves treasures that will come back to you in consciousness of duty well done...things that, having given away freely, you yet possess."

Aging, sidelined, disarmed, Rene Caisse found her resistance to stress lessening. In the relative anonymity of North Bay, away from the headlines, the Commissions, the endless river of cancer sufferers, her nerves succumbed, and she spiraled downward in a nervous collapse. She would later use the term 'breakdown' to describe her collapse. In short it may very well have been that 'delirium of the deep' that overwhelms divers when they come to the surface too fast. It was decompression not depression that overtook Rene Caisse once life became 'normal'.

It would not last long. Soon, Charles McGaughey, having developed 'the old man's friend' at the very young age of 57, died of pneumonia in North Bay. Rene made the decision to return to live among her friends in Bracebridge.

CHAPTER TWO

ALL ABOUT YIELDING

> "Short days ago we lived, loved, laughed, saw sunset's glow. But now..."
>
> John McCrae, *In Flanders Fields*

In 1948, Rene Caisse was almost 60 when she crossed the bridge into town. Home once more. A glance uphill to the left after leaving the bridge would verify that the once upon a time clinic still stood overseeing Dominion Street. No lights in the window.

The nuclear age was three years old. Figure skating was all the rage.

Barbara Anne Scott of Canada won Olympic gold in St. Moritz. Twelve skaters yet had to perform when the blonde Canadian teenager left the ice but the crowd had already crowned Barbara Anne as the golden girl to replace Sonia Henie as the queen of the ice in the eyes of the world.

Perhaps there should be an Olympics for cancer cures. They had a form of Olympics for poets in France. Third prize was a bronze rose. Second prize was a silver rose. First prize was a real rose. For a Cancer Cure Olympics third place would get a bronze medal from the CMA, second a silver, the first place winner would get to shake the hand of a patient getting well.

Memories of old battles, pressures, controversies, of the faces of her countless patients must have crowded her memory, competing for her attentions with news of the rapidly changing world. Like 90% of other Canadian homes, she used radio to be kept abreast of the turmoil in India, the birth pains of Israel, the ominous talk of Russia getting the bomb. Now and then medicine made news.

In March, the Ontario Government announced a $100,000 research foundation grant to be applied in conjunction with Alcoholics Anonymous. The United Nations adopted the Universal declaration of Human Rights. Women in Canada, by government policy, would now have equal rights to employment and equal pay. Interesting concept. Wonder what the nursing world thinks of that?

Just before Christmas, margarine which had been banned in Canada since 1886 was made legal. The dairy industry was upset. But the Supreme Court ruled that the nameless, faceless designers of the Dairy Industry Act which banned margarine had fashioned a human construct that was ultra vires, that is to say, illegal, because it was outside of Parliament's powers. Five days before Christmas the first margarine went on sale in Vancouver. Doubtless they had portrayed margarine as a danger to mankind. Doubtless they would have tested it on mice for thirty years rather than see it cut into their control over the dairy industry. Doubtless they had seen margarine as a threat to their own job security, but most importantly as a threat to their power to fashion human constructs, ultra vires or otherwise, that would cement their hammerlock on dairy products and the lives of consumers.

McKenzie King handed over the reins of power to Louis St. Laurent. Newfoundland agreed to enter Confederation. The two events were not connected.

September 23, 1949, President Truman announced that the Soviet Union had exploded their first atomic bomb. Nuclear fallout and the effects of radiation fueled the panic that launched the bomb shelter era. The single force the cancer industry, after 50 years of research, had been able to bring to bear on mutating tumors was now the cause of world-wide terror. Overnight the world understood that radiation meant mutilation and death.

June 25, 1951, North Korea invaded South Korea. News reel footage of the effects of atomic fallout on the survivors of the bomb in Hiroshima and Nagasaki were replayed in people's minds even before they became regular viewing on television. Science fiction portrayed survivors of bomb shelters staggering over burned out top soil with tumors eating up their faces and skulls. No place to hide, was the message. Ray guns gave radiation a new life, film writers actually getting it right, that radiation killed. Far from recognizing however that the killing force had been here all along, an entire phenomenon was launched to answer society's frantic demand for some explanation of the new peril: the UFO culture swept across the United States, Canada and the world. Still, as fantasies of extra-terrestrial invaders piercing the solitude of earth, raping it of its resources and obliterating every man, woman and child, spun out of control, the real invasion continued, cancer piercing the body's immune system and consuming everything in sight.

In August, Canada announced it would send an expeditionary force to fight under the United Nations' banner in Korea. Bracebridge mothers whose sons had been too young to be swept up in the 39-45 War now felt real peril enter their lives.

1951, in London, Ontario, the world's first Cobalt radiotherapy unit for treatment of cancer, developed in Canada by Harold Johns and others, was installed at the Victoria Hospital.

1952 brought a new Queen of England and the Korean armistice. Observing life instead of saving it was a tame exercise, at best, in contrast to all the years of struggle. Then 1952 brought a reminder that Rene Caisse and Essiac had not been forgotten by the world.

A letter arrived from Rome. Soon afterward another, even more urgent, from Godfrey A.P.V. Winter Baumgarten, imploring her help in the case of someone suffering from cancer, someone known throughout the world, someone who not too long ago had set Europe on its ear, was the darling of the media and continually captured the eye of the whole world in everything she did. The opportunity to treat this person would result in instantaneous world wide acknowledgment of Essiac. The sufferer in question was the 32 year old wife of Juan Peron, the dictator of Argentina.

They now called Eva Duarte, 'Evita', affectionate, intimate term meaning Little Eva. To the media she was Evita Duarte de Peron. To the Peronistas of Argentina she was Senora La Presidente. To international diplomats she was the First Lady of La Casa Rosada, the pink stuccoed equivalent of the White House. She was also, according to Rene's information, now known as Evelyn Paro, and was waiting in Duluth Michigan, for Rene Caisse to make contact.

Argentina's First Lady? In Duluth, Michigan? Waiting for the nurse from Bracebridge? What did Rene Caisse make of it all? It had to do with money and power and media prominence. It had to do with a remarkable woman who had lived life her way and taken Argentina by storm. So much was dependent on Evita Peron. Was she not the single greatest patron of the poor in South America?

Was it not rumored that she was practically bankrupting the government by giving out handfuls of money to the unemployed and the hungry? Was she not the patron of the hundreds of thousands of 'shirtless ones' in Argentina's workforce?

Her every move was monitored and reported by the press. What a coup it would be to have the world know that she was cured of cancer at the age of 32 by Essiac! Juan Peron would see to it that the whole world knew the cause of his wife's survival. He was known to be designing monuments to himself and his friends for a futuristic landscape of Argentina. Was Rene Caisse destined to be immortalized on some hill top overlooking Buenos Aires?

Rene never went to Duluth. The siren call of hundreds of thousands of 'shirtless ones' waving their arms in jubilation at Evita's survival could not compare to the gesture of those CNR rail men in Capreol who raised a dollar at a time to send Tony Bazuk to Bracebridge and to Rene Caisse in the mid Thirties, and not all the arm waving in the world could be more meaningful than Annie Bonner's right arm, the arm that Dr. Leonardo said was dead, being raised under Annie's own steam, to testify at the Cancer Commission of 1939 that Essiac had restored her arm to life.

Fame and fortune, awaiting her in Duluth, did not lure Rene Caisse out of Bracebridge. The decision not to go and be swept away by the high drama and hoopla merely reinforced the reality that every aspect of her life over the years confirmed - that she had no interest in gaining financially from Essiac. From the mid 1930's she had withstood offers from scientific agencies or individual humanitarians as well as entrepreneurs. She remained fiercely protective of it, determined that it would never be exploited for money, insisting always that it belonged to suffering humanity as a whole.

But by 1952 it did not belong to mankind as a whole. Essiac remained as it had always been, the secret of Rene Caisse. Critics inside and outside of the medical profession continued to challenge her on the point, if she believed it belonged to everyone, why not reveal her herbal formula?

Her response never varied.

"I have always been and am still willing to turn over my formula to the medical association anytime that they will assure me that it will be used to help suffering humanity, and that it will not be shelved in favor of present day methods of treatments..."

She remained convinced that 'certain vested interests' were dead set against her treatment becoming known. The conspiracy theory that had insinuated itself into her world view could not have been lessened by the political and social climate of the day. Her past near arrests and the constant threat of actual imprisonment was still ever present in her mind. It was after all, the McCarthy era, when fear of communism had been the tool whereby the powerful had found the means to frighten every man and woman in America out of their wits as a means perhaps of frightening them out of their rights.

Throughout the entire run of the McCarthy era when witch hunting had reached heights unknown in even medieval times, Rene Caisse was all too well aware that the Health Department was keeping track of her activities. They knew that she was treating some patients out of her Bracebridge home.

In 1953, Canada had 8,000 polio cases with 481 deaths to deal with, yet they kept an eye on Bracebridge. That year, the American researcher Jonas Salk reported to the U.S. National Foundation Immunizing Committee confirmation of his polio vaccine, yet they kept an eye on Bracebridge.

In 1956, the CMA journal announced that kissing might be responsible for the increase in mononucleosis. Mono became linked in the public's mind with pigeons, earning the nickname 'pigeon's disease'. Nobody asked who had been the first person to kiss a pigeon and bring the disease into society but netheless people were running away from pigeons in the street, teachers warning tots not to feed them. And still they kept an eye on Bracebridge.

In 1957, the Cannought Laboratories in Toronto announced their quadruple vaccine against polio, diptheria, tetanus and whooping cough. And they kept their eye on Bracebridge.

By 1958, the powers that be made one more attempt at forcing the Bracebridge nurse into the open. The secretary for the Commission for the Investigation of Cancer Remedies, in a letter dated May 29, 1958, one C.J. Telfer, wrote to the Minister of Health, Dr. Mackinnon Philips.

It said, "...At a meeting of the Commission a letter was read from Miss Caisse, the nurse from Bracebridge who refused many years ago to divulge the formula which she then and apparently still is using in the treatment of cancer. The Commission feels no action should be taken by them, but directed the matter be brought to your attention in case you might wish to refer this one also to the College of Physicians and Surgeons."

The Premier of the Province of Ontario was Leslie Frost. He advised Rene by letter to give the Commission 'the details of your methods' so the Commission could give them 'a thorough analysis'.

In her response to Frost, in a letter to the deputy Minister of health, Dr. W. G. Brown to whom Frost had directed her, Rene stated, "I told Dr. Banting, Dr. Noble and Dr. B.T. McGie 20 years ago, that when the medical world would give me some assurance that this treatment would be used by them in the treatment of cancer, I would be willing to give them the formula.

"They would not give me this assurance, so I decided that if they did not know what I was using they would not be in a position to condemn it. I have therefore kept my own counsel."

Dr. McPhedran of the College of Physicians and Surgeons ordered her to stop treating patients at her home. When she did not he sent his policemen to arrest her. It was like old times.

"I'm glad," she wrote,"that when Dr. McPhedran sent his policemen here to arrest me, that I had not too many patients to turn away. I closed my clinic years ago, but patients came begging for treatment at my home, and I could not turn them away."

Then with spirited irony she added, "Now the onus is on the medical profession. I have to turn them away."

Though she was not prosecuted she remained under surveillance.

There is a secret about yielding. It becomes not more probable but less so as a person ages. By 1959, Rene Caisse was nearing seventy years of age. She had been shepherding Essiac for 37 years, keeping the wolves away from the flock and away from the formula. Anyone attempting to lure her into the open at this stage in her life simply did not know her history.

In 1959, the Brusch Medical Center in Cambridge succeeded in bringing Rene Caisse to their laboratories, where they had been studying quantities of Essiac that Rene had sent to them from Canada in response to their request. Dr. Charles Brusch appointed 18 doctors to supervise the famous nurse's experimentations when she arrived there to treat terminal cancer patients. And of course, there were more mice.

A new name, a new star was on everybody's lips, that senator from Massachussetts who was about to lead the Democratic Party to the White House, John Fitzgerald Kennedy. Kennedy's personal physician was the same Dr. Charles Brusch with whom Rene was now working. Once again the proximity to a famous name, one that would have made the letters 'Essiac' as familiar to American households as JFK was available to her.

Within only three months The Brusch Medical Center concluded about Essiac that, "Clinically on patients suffering from pathologically proven cancer, it reduces pain and causes a recession in the growth; patients have gained weight and shown an improvement in their general health."

They did not say it was a cure. Would they have had she revealed the formula? She did not yield. Even so Dr. Brusch himself remained one of Essiac's foremost advocates and would resort to it himself when he was later diagnosed with cancer. He gave it full credit for his cure.

Brusch had studies on Essiac conducted in four American laboratories as well as one in Canada, all of whom supported his conclusion that it was a remedy for cancer. Brusch's greatest regret was that Kennedy was assassinated before Brusch could encourage him to lend his influence to the promotion of Essiac in the medical community.

The death of Kennedy gave conspiracy theorists worldwide a new symbol for their paranoia, 'the man on the grassy knoll', the epitome of the nameless, faceless oppressor. The fact that Rene Caisse had seen a 'conspiracy' against her treatment in the cancer industry does not mean she was paranoid. A person who has been threatened with jail has reason to be cautious, to weigh the sincerity of those trying to imprison her. There was no 'man on the grassy knoll' in Rene Caisse's view of the medical establishment. She would have been the first to state that every one who opposed her in the Commission hearings over the years were men of good intent with no dark purpose, no ill will. It was that illusive thing called 'power' that was her adversary, most especially directed at her from its base of operations within the mid level bureaucracy of medical institutions and government. It has ever been so when power is about to be lost, that those wielding it are driven to destroy their adversaries to protect their grip on their share of power. The 'man on the grassy knoll' became a household phrase because America interpreted Kennedy as a threat to certain vested interests and those vested interests felt it best to fix him in their cross hairs.

The grassy knoll gave America a reason to smoulder.

Rene Caisse, both in her private and professional life, though all who knew her would testify that she was nobody's fool, gave the benefit of the doubt even to her detractors. That was the means by which she overcame bitterness and prevented the anger from getting a foothold in her psyche. It is noteworthy that throughout it all she remained basically healthy.

"Healing is how you live your life."

As they had on previous occasions with other sponsors, bureaucrats in the cancer industry exerted pressure on the Brusch Center and the number of patients made available for testing petered out. Rene returned home to Bracebridge the formula still intact, still solely in her possession. Decades of frustration bore down upon her when she returned. The desperation that had so often overtaken suffering cancer victims had finally overtaken the resolve of the incorruptible, unshakable nurse. In a move completely inconsistent with her long and remarkable career, she threw out 27,000 treatments of Essiac.

There is a certain theatricality to this gesture that echoes of previous moments in her life: finding Mrs. Gilrouth's diagnosis at the last moment, allowing her photo to be printed on the Hepburn election flyers with the reminder of his promise to voters emblazoned, chasing a patient down the street to return to him money he left for compensation for his treatment, threatening to close the clinic, then the filling of the ballroom at the Royal York with 387 supporters, closing the clinic. In each of these dramatic moments, Rene Caisse was writing chapter headings to the story of her life. She knew that history would be kinder, gentler in its judgment of her than the Cancer Commission had been. It was directly to posterity that she was directing her message in each of these gestures. She never hit a false note in her whole adventure, and history would see that she was capable of the large gesture to emphasize that point. In all of these turning points in her life we see confirmation of the efficacy of her treatment, for, it was her total faith in it that directed her in her moments of high drama on the world stage.

Throwing out 27,000 treatments of Essiac was a gesture history would use to underline her absolute refusal to yield to corruption or persuasion. Van Gogh's detractor's like to say that if Vincent had been truly serious he would have severed his painting hand instead of his ear but that would have deprived the world of his genius. Destroying 27,000 treatments of the herbal formula did not deny the world the treatment. She still retained the formula. Nevertheless, it must have been a liberating act, like turning the clock to the wall that had monitored so many years of waiting, of restriction, of responsibility. She still had the formula, after all.

Dr. Philip Merker of the Memorial Sloan-Kettering Institute and the National Cancer Institute of the United States wanted to test Essiac but insisted Rene Caisse reveal the formula. She did not yield. A final chapter was written, however, between 1973 and 1976 when Sloan-Kettering proceeded, with her cooperation, to test on mice the material she sent them. She refused to send the written formula, then lost interest.

Time was indeed passing quickly. She was now 87 years of age.

For decades she had challenged the medical establishment and government bureaucracy, refusing to reveal the Essiac formula to medical authorities, scientific researchers, or business interests.

She had always insisted, as the price to get her to reveal the formula, a guarantee that there would be official public recognition of the merits of Essiac by governing bodies, that Essiac would remain available to people who needed it and that it would not vanish into laboratories for animal testing. Since no one would give that guarantee she refused all offers.

Until October, 1977.

The Resperin Corporation of Toronto was a familiar entity to Rene Caisse. At one time they had made an offer to Rene, to test the product and to place her on a weekly fee schedule during the testing. The offer was not overly generous in terms of the amount offered. It was understood by everyone that a nurse who had once turned down a million dollars for her formula could not be bought. The fee offered was a token of acknowledgment of her ownership of Essiac. She refused in any case. Refusal had become almost a habit.

Take up our quarrel with the foe...

In 1977, Rene Caisse was approaching 90 years of age. It might be forgiven a nurse with Rene's history of never yielding to pressure, that she might enjoy knowing that the nameless, faceless power hungry bureaucrats who had tried relentlessly to break her spirit, and when they could not do that to slander her character and vilify her name, were still nameless and faceless, while she, in her small modest home in Bracebridge had maintained the love of her patients and the respect of the giants of the medical profession. Nevertheless, it was time for younger hearts to press the fight.

It might also be forgiven her, if she waited with something akin to personal and professional pride as some of those same professionals, on a beautiful northern October day, were heading north to Bracebridge in a cavalcade of automobiles, to receive from her hand the formula she had so long secreted from pubic view.

The leaves of Muskoka hold nothing back in autumn. September confronts the eye with colors not seen since Creation: reds, hot yellows, ochre, leathery black maple confounding the eye with purple, colors one can taste and savor long after the leaves have fallen.

By October some leaves still lingered though most had dropped to surrender the horizon to the muted mauve of a perpetual gloaming. A boy in the Fifties seated along this highway north would have been able to identify the make of each automobile from a half mile off at the first flash of a chrome bumper or a tail fin. But by 1977, cars had started to all look the same, heavy, ponderous, cumbersome on the turns, faceless, nameless with nothing to distinguish them one from another as they streamed elegantly toward the famous bridge of the famous town but the flags fluttering on aerials.

The wind of the river gave them a good whipping as they rolled sedately into view, miniature flags of Canada, of Ontario, officialdom fluttering into town for a visit long overdue, arriving at last at fortress Bracebridge where the famous nurse had been protected and defended and supported if not like a princess in a walled city, then at least a favored daughter.

It was a town with a moat of its own, the protective Muskoka River running rapidly through the abrupt cut between the ascending slope of the approach and the hill beyond on which stood the town. It had a drawbridge of sorts, although it didn't draw or move up or swing left or right, the famous silver bridge that had been the sign to so many sufferers that they had arrived at the doorway to all their hopes. Beyond the bridge, the town climbed and crowned a miniature hill, much the way castles and battlements of old chose the high ground for safety. In the center of Bracebridge is the office of the Bracebridge Examiner whose editor Ted Britton, fittingly, had written his doctoral thesis on The Medieval Social Ville, long before moving to Bracebridge.

That autumn Britton placed his newspaper at Rene Caisse's disposal so that she could tell "...her own story about her struggle to have Essiac recognized as a cancer treatment."

It was a chance to have the last word, the very thing the medical establishment had denied her.

He interviewed the world famous nurse at length, writing up the story without editorial comment or changes. She asked him to print the story posthumously so that "...she would at least have her say on the whole Essiac controversy."

He added, "In this way, at least, the people of Rene Caisse's home town will know what she thought of the single issue which dominated most of her adult life."

The flags fluttered through town, the long somber limousines turning to the right of the main street of town to roll slowly along Hiram Street until they came to a stop before the small brick home of Rene Caisse.

To you from failing hands we throw the torch

What thoughts played in Rene's mind as she watched Pauline McKibbon, Lieutenant Governor of Ontario, disembark and walk up the driveway to her door? For over half of the 20th Century she had withstood insult, libel, slander, threats of imprisonment. Throughout she had refused to be annihilated by the crushing hurt that was her constant companion and only wage for her service to the suffering. She never grew bitter. Bitterness is a disease of the mind that can consume the heart. It is a sickness that must be healed and, 'Healing is how you live you life." The jewel in her crown was that she never charged, but rather accepted donations only, for any of her life-long service to the sick.

But the time had come to hand over her formula to somebody

she clearly believed had the ability to get Essiac approved as a cancer treatment. Resperin Corporation met all the requirements to make Essaic accessible and inexpensive to all.

Be yours to hold it high

That October day on Hiram Street in 1977, 55 years after she had listened to the story of campfires and gold fever from the Englishwoman Mrs. A., Rene Caisse signed over the sole proprietary rights to the Essiac formula and trademark for the grand sum of $1.00 Canadian. It was a singular act of charity by a Canadian woman whose whole life had been one prolonged act of service to the sick.

If ye break faith with us who die

At her side, attesting to the fact that the formula had never before been revealed to anyone other than Resperin was Dr. Charles Brusch of Cambridge, Mass., official witness to the signing of the contract.

CHAPTER THREE

YESTERDAY

Eight thousand years after the Tyrell Sea began to shrink into what is now Hudson's Bay, and the retreating glaciers had scraped clean the surface of the great mineral shield hanging like a bib around the neck of the Bay, an Indian stepped into the light of an evening campfire and cured a woman of cancer. For eight thousand years, even along the margins of the slowly retreating glaciers, his ancestors had been born, lived and died. When history began to be recorded the offspring of those hardy nomads were identified as the Cree who hunted and fished the rivers flowing into Hudson's Bay and the Ojibway who worked the rivers flowing into Lake Superior.

It was then and remains today a land of yesterday. Robert Rennison recorded his thoughts on it in 1888.

'I entered a land of yesterday. The twilight of the romance of the Hudson's Bay company still hovered over Ontario's backdoor. The Dominion Government sent down occasional surveyors. The Indians were left alone...There were only two outside interests, the old Company that came for fur, and the Missionaries who remembered that Indians had souls." [1]

A few years after Rennison wrote those words, an Englishwoman who discovered she had breast cancer was shown the cure by an unnamed Ojibway who showed her specific botanicals growing wild in the soil of the Shield, plants with a very high mineral content. The identity of these herbs, where to find them, when to harvest them, in what proportions and for what length of time to brew them, were passed on by the Englishwoman to a young 34 year old nurse in the Sisters of Providence Hospital in Haileybury, Ontario, in 1922. The notes written down by the nurse that day became the secret of Essiac, the name given the formula by the young woman Rene Caisse.

That formula is with us today because Rene Caisse devoted her entire life to protecting it and keeping it out of the hands of those who would exploit it and even outlaw it. In 1977, one year before her death she revealed the proprietary formula for the first time to the representatives of the Resperin Corporation of Toronto.

The Herbal Formula

"It was so simple, I never thought anyone would believe it," Rene Caisse once said.

Chances are, unless you are living in the center of a concrete city, you could put this book down and without walking perhaps 1000 paces in any direction from your house, find one or more of four main botanicals that have been used for centuries in countries all over the world to detoxify the body, cleanse the blood, and restore health to the cells. The four main botanicals of the formula that have been restoring health to many thousands of people worldwide since 1922, are *Burdock Root, Slippery Elm, Sheep Sorrel and Indian Rhubarb.*

"I want this clearly understood," Rene said in 1977, "I did not get my treatment from an Indian. In fact I never saw a real Indian in my life."

This tongue in cheek dismantling of the sentiment that all the world's ailments could be resolved by native wisdom may have had as its oblique purpose to comfort those who later would question whether or not the four main herbs in Essiac were in the original recipe given to the Englishwoman. Burdock Root and Slippery Elm are known to have been available to and used by the indigenous people of the region throughout history, but Indian Rhubarb Root and Sheep Sorrel were not. If these latter botanicals were in fact Rene Caisse's formula, then it justifies her life long proprietorship of Essiac.

Rene would say, "One has just to look at a dirty roadside in the spring and see how nature covers it up with beautiful greens and flowers, to know that nature supplies everything to make life beautiful and healthy."

"If nature will do this for a dirty roadside, is it not natural to think that it will also supply the things necessary to make the body (made in the image and likeness of God) healthy and happy?"[2]

With the hindsight of fifty years experience she could express herself freely on the cancer industry.

"The cancer society has been in existence for over fifty years and everyone donates to their support, hoping each year that they will find something beneficial in the treatment of this dread disease, which is claiming so many of our loved ones, but up to date they know not the cause nor the cure."[3]

On the origins of cancer growth she said, "Malignant cells form and feed upon the healthy ones. I believe there is an interchange of substance between the malignant cells and the healthy cells of the body; malignant cells absorbing from the healthy cells, that which is required for their growth and development, while they throw off into the human body, something which emaciates and destroys it. In this dreadful growth, the healthy tissue is destroyed until finally a living destructive organ dominates and spreads its evil along without resistance."[4]

Dr. Paavo Airola: "The primary and ultimate cause of cancer is lowered or broken down resistance of the body's own defense mechanism against the singular or combined physical, chemical, emotional and environmental stresses."[5]

The corrective device for setting the body right again is in nature itself.

The first botanical is Burdock (Arctium Lappa): in 1966 Hungarian researchers discovered antitumor activity in Burdock. The Burdock Root contains as its principal ingredient and main curative agent the oil inulin, a powerful immune modulator that attaches to the surface of white cells and makes them work better. Inulin is the vital and active agent in the metabolism of carbohydrates.[6] It inhibits the growth of harmful bacteria.[7] Burdock also contains benzaldehyde, a substance which has significant anti-cancer effects in humans.

Years before the HIV crisis, Burdock Root's inulin had already been proven to be effective on the immune system. The Kawasi School of Medicine at Nagoya University in Okayama, Japan, found Burdock to be effective in reducing cell mutation. They called it the Burdock-Factor. The oil, they determined, is found to be active against HIV. Containing vitamin A and selenium, and another broad array of minerals, it is vital source of nutrition strength.[8]

The current astronomical costs of medications for HIV patients, raises the specter once more of what the AIDS industry, already a multi-billion dollar business, would initiate against Essiac were it to be acknowledged as a means of restoring HIV patients to health. Rene Caisse had already fought much of the battle for HIV sufferers by protecting her Essiac with her life.

The second botanical - Sheep Sorrel (Rumex Acetosella). This vinegar plant has been a staple of folk medicine throughout history. As early as the 1740's its use in the treatment of cancer was acknowledged when "legislation was introduced in Williamsburg, Virginia, to allow one Mary Johnson to use Sheep Sorrel for that purpose. [9] Sheep Sorrel contains silicon, is rich in minerals, vitamins: "the fresh juice of the sorrel leaves nourishes all the glands in the body."[10] It nourishes the glandular system, and strengthens the myellin sheath that protects the nerves.

"Chlorophyl, the green pigment in the leaves and stems of Sheep Sorrel, is 'concentrated sun power'. It closely resembles hemoglobin, the red pigment in human blood, but has as its center a magnesium atom whereas hemoglobin is constructed around the iron atom, and both carry oxygen to every cell of the organism."[11]

Premium quality herbs and exact ratios are vital. The correct ratios are vitally important. Source of the herbs and where they are grown is of paramount importance because of the absence of quality control standards in this field in North America. Harvesting times are vitally important. Indian Rhubarb Root must be six years old while Burdock Root must be from first year plants.

Rene often called cancer a 'glandular disease'.

"I believe," said Rene, "there is a gland to supply us with the secretion to resist the malignant cells and it is active in some people and not in others. This gland has not been discovered by medical science as yet, but when it is, the cause of cancer will be known.

"Cancer generally follows the line of least resistance and does not cause pain or even inconvenience in its early stages, until it has invaded an organ or nerve center. It may be slow in development and in such cases is most deceptive and difficult to discover or feel. It may develop rapidly and make itself felt early, when it can be fairly easily diagnosed and treated. A slow growing cancer may not bother a person for years, until it affects a vital organ. In its rapid growth, however, a few months of progress may make it too late for the surgeon's knife and then deep X-ray therapy may only scatter it to other parts, while radium drives it in, instead of out, and burns the surrounding tissue. I believe that radium, used in too heavy doses, is the prolific cause of further cancer in the destroyed burnt tissue.

"Once the cancer gets into the glands to any extent, medical science accepts defeat. In many cases, infected internal glands cannot be treated by any of the above-mentioned methods. The same applies to all the vital organs. If the affected part can, in its infancy, be cut out by surgery before the malignancy starts shooting out its fine spider-web like tentacles, a cure can and is sometimes affected. Once, however, the cancer becomes active and starts to travel to any extent, as it does along the line of least resistance, following its insidious relentless course, any destructive agency applied to the human body can only do more harm.

"Essiac...supplies a deficiency of a secretion ordinarily supplied to the human body by a gland which we call 'Gland XOX'. Some people are born with a predisposition to cancer with a non-functioning XOX gland and the slightest bruise or destruction of cells will cause the disease to become active.

"Essiac given to people in health is helpful in the fact that it is a blood purifier and will stimulate the XOX gland to do its work before there is a chance of the malignant cells invading the body. This gland should supply the body with a secretion which is resistant to cancer tissue. The lack of this secretion allows the malignant cells to prey upon and invade the healthy cells and take control of the human body, growing and multiplying until the invasion of the malignant cells into the vital organs takes place, stopping the functioning of these organs and causing death.

"The deficiency cannot be supplied from the 'outside', it must be supplied through the blood stream and Essiac ... supplies this resistive element. Then the XOX gland starts functioning normally, secreting into the living cells the substance required to resist the onslought of the malignant cells and thus restores health to the human body. If this was not the case, patients would have to take Essiac for the rest of their lives as they do with insulin for diabetes."[12]

The third botanical is Slippery Elm, (Ulmus Fulva). Long accepted as one of the best known herbal remedies, the inner bark of this North American tree, is rich in calcium, magnesium and organ feeding vitamins A,B,C, K. It contains beta-sitosterol and a polysaccharide that also demonstrate anti-tumor activity, contains large amounts of tannins and mucilages, is active against sore throats, dissolves mucous deposits in tissues, glands and nerve channels, ulcers and as an anti-inflammatory for the digestive system. Its slippery characteristic lubricates bones and joints.[13]

"The treatment (Essiac) goes to the seat of the trouble no matter where it is," said Rene, " whether internally or on the surface, and gives to the healthy cells, the strength to resist the demands of malignant cells for the substance upon which the malignancy thrives, thus causing a recession of the malignant cells from the healthy cells, which have become stronger."[14]

The fourth botanical is Indian Rhubarb Root (Rheum Officianale). It is rich in iron, harvested in the form of a thick root, acts as a gentle laxative, purging the liver and the body of wastes and toxic build-up and waste.

The American Office of Technology Assessment found Indian Rhubarb Root and Sorrel both contain aloe, catechin and rehin which have demonstrated anti-tumor activity in animal tests. Can be used internally and externally.

"Essiac attacks the disease from the 'inside'. It sets up a resistance and cuts off the supply of the substances in the human body upon which the malignant cells thrive and multiply, causing the malignant cells to regress within themselves and giving to the healthy cells, strength to rebuild themselves. Medical science calls these malignant cells dead cells. They are more alive and aggressive than any cells in the human body."[15]

Rene adds, "I do not believe that cancer is caused by viruses, but I can readily believe that a malignant mass can create viruses and that is where the interchange of substances between the malignant cells and the healthy cells takes place. The malignant cells take from the healthy cells, and in the exchange throw off viruses into the healthy cells, in order to weaken and destroy them. I feel sure that if viruses are discovered, it will be in this area.

"As for cancer being hereditary, my experience with many thousands of patients tells me that it is in some cases. I do not mean that one inherits the actual growth, but that one can inherit a predisposition to the disease and any destruction of cells in these people will set up a malignant growth. However, at the present time, there are babies being born with malignancy, of parents who have no history of cancer at all.

"It is reasonable to conclude that no destructive agent can be successfully applied to eradicate a cancerous growth which has more power in its wildly growing cells in a living organism and their destructive ability, than the resistant ability of any organ in the human body. The malignancy is born of some freak of nature which has reversed the process of renewing wasting tissue and building up new healthy cells.

"Although not admitted by Medical science, cancer is, in my opinion, both contagious and hereditary in some cases. The rapid spread of this dread disease could not be caused by any other means.

"It has been found in post-mortems that individuals have had cancer during their lives without knowing of its existence and the cancer had increased to the extent that all that remained was the evidence that destructive work had at one time been done and stopped. Nature had either supplied the body with the resistance or more probably, the human system ceased to supply the malignant cells with the material vital to its existence.

"The human body cannot stand the havoc and destruction caused by any external irritating or lethal agent such as radiation, which is strong enough to destroy living cancer, and must consequently destroy the living tissue, including the healthy tissue.

"Unfortunately there are few physicians who can diagnose cancer, or very few symptoms to warn the individual or the doctor, in the majority of cases. Especially in many internal afflictions there are few, if any, noticeable symptoms and in the majority of these cases, the disease is too well established or rooted before the doctor or his patient even suspect its presence.

"Today, the only remedies in general practice and recognized by the medical profession, as the result of the above efforts, are surgery, radium and deep X-ray therapy. It is quite apparent... that surgery, radium and deep X-ray are not the answers."[16]

Ted Britton, Editor and Publisher of the Bracebridge Examiner, in a statement accompanying the publication in the Bracebridge Examiner of Rene's own story in her own words added, "Rene always felt strongly that certain vested interests were opposed to her work and this comes across repeatedly...Whether or not a conspiracy of sorts has worked against Essiac and other possible cancer cures remains to be proven in fact, but Nurse Caisse certainly felt the cards were always stacked against her."[17]

It was big business the nurse from Bracebridge was up against. The total cost for cancer in 1991 was $100 billion. [18]

"Indeed," wrote Britton, "she believed that life could be made very difficult for anyone who suggested that there might be a simple safe cure for cancer. Certainly, if one reads Rene's account of what she went through in trying to have Essiac recognized, it is at least understandable that she felt there were very powerful and influential forces working against her." (19)

"...if some simple and inexpensive replacement for chemotherapy for the treatment of cancer were found tomorrow," said Dr. Barry Lynes, " all US medical schools would teeter on the verge of bankruptcy so integral a part of their hospital revenue is oncology."[20]

That the cancer industry is not a charity, that it is big business, was the cornerstone of Rene Caisse's refusal for over half a century to yield up the secret of her famous herbal formula. In doing so she saved it from oblivion.

Requiem

Rene Caisse died, the day after Christmas Day, 1978.

"A Requiem Mass was held for Rene Caisse at St. Joseph's Catholic Church (in Bracebridge) at 11:00 AM last Friday. Nurse Caisse, who died at South Muskoka Memorial Hospital on December 26th, suffered a broken leg in a fall at her Hiram St. home five weeks ago, from which she never recovered.

"When she died, Rene was 91 and had reached the summit of her professional career as the developer of Essiac, a herbal tea said by many to be a positive benefit in the treatment of cancer." -Ted Britton, Editor, Bracebridge Examiner.

Rene Caisse, herself, never actually called it a cure for cancer. What she did say about it is a perfect summation of her life and her career.

"I treated cancer with Essiac ... for many decades successfully. I am a nurse, not a doctor, therefore I always made sure that every case was diagnosed by a qualified physician and as often as possible administered treatment under the observation of doctors.

"Essiac is a herbal treatment ...and is quite harmless even to a well person. I have hoped to prove that it is a preventive medication. As a rule, patients were presented by their doctors after everything known to medical science had been used and failed. Even in the most advanced cases I was able to stop hemorrhaging, relieve pain and prolong life.

"Medical science has tried all of the unnatural means at its disposal to combat this dread disease with little or no results. Nature has supplied the need to combat the disease."

Her legacy is a life lived in the practical application of the four cardinal virtues. She exhibited wisdom. She remained temperate through intemperate times. From these attributes she drew the courage to struggle for justice for cancer sufferers.

Cicero extols such qualities as the leadership ideal for which every man should strive.

"Each man should so conduct himself that fortitude appears in labors and dangers: temperance in foregoing pleasures: prudence in the choice between good and evil: justice in giving every man his own."

Add to that, that in a war-filled world in a century where a lot of people believe and a lot of people trust yet still manage to produce a society built on the worship of self, her life progressed in three stages from faith, through hope, to a most singular act of charity and the conclusion is inescapable. Rene Caisse was a three act play in a two act world.

Today, the Rene Caisse Memorial Room maintained by the Bracebridge Historical Society, stands next to the town edge of the bridge that had been the insignia of hope for so many cancer sufferers for so many years. To find it, just cross the bridge and turn right.

AFTERWORD

The drama of Rene Caisse and Essiac are integrated into the psyche of Bracebridge like silken threads in a fine weave. When her name comes up in conversation with a resident of Bracebridge, more often than not, a look is exchanged, that-moment-of-recognition-look one might expect to see from a connoisseur caressing the fabric of a prize quilt, the look that denotes appreciation of quality. One more life of quality is Rene Caisse's legacy to the town that supported her.

Just as there are people at every county fair who will pass by a fine quilt without giving it a touch, one can still encounter a small number on Manitoba Street, Bracebridge's main street, mostly from the younger generation, who do not know they are a player strutting their stuff on the very stage where one of the most endearing adventures in Canadian history was enacted. Such is the patchwork of which quilts and towns are made.

The patchwork of volunteerism, one might say, is what keeps a town warm. Towns are made warm by historical memory. Museums. Libraries. Exhibits. And then there are the people who carry history in their heart, their soul, their eyes.

In the course of researching Bridge of Hope, a magical serendipity surfaced. I kept meeting all the right people. I would set out for the library to research someone and find myself sitting beside them at the Rene Caisse collection, head off to Woodchester Villa to see and touch some of the artifacts from Rene's life and be asked to help carry in some new find, go searching for the old barbershop where Joseph Caisse cut a few thousand miles of the town's hair and be shown through the attic by the woman who nursed Rene in her last years, go to the Town Hall to ask where I could find Ken Veitch only to discover I was talking to him.

Then there was the mystery, a fine silken thread indeed, that continually surfaced throughout this small town weave. The mystery was that even people who did not respond knowingly to the name Rene Caisse knew that the name was inextricably linked with another name. Whether at the library, the Rene Caisse Room at Woodchester Villa, on Manitoba Street or at Town Hall, the name kept reappearing. That name was Mary McPherson.

Mary McPherson was a lifelong friend of Rene Caisse. As a volunteer working alongside Rene Caisse, she saw the decades of hope and disappointment come and go. She is the single most vital link with the story of Rene Caisse. She lives in Bracebridge and is considered the rightful custodian of the Rene Caisse legend. The desire to meet her, however, was tempered by the fact that she had been just recently hospitalized. It was determined then to accomplish as much as possible on the book while hoping an opportunity would present itself to meet her.

That opportunity came through Ken Veitch. Ken can quite fairly be called the unofficial historian of the Rene Caisse story. His contribution to this rendering of Rene's life began with a guided tour through the old barbershop of Rene's father, continued throughout the search for photographic documentation, orchestrated introductions to Mayor Scott Northmore, the Town Council, and Don McVittie, relative and enthusiast of Rene Caisse, and ultimately produced what without him may have remained unattainable — a meeting with Mary McPherson.

In a hospitality room in the South Muskoka Memorial Hospital, I finally got to meet Mary McPherson. Together with Ken Veitch, Don McVittie and T.P. Maloney, President of Essiac Canada International, I had the pleasure of spending several hours with the woman who had been there through it all and could relive with a word or a phrase incidents that are part of the legend of Essiac.

Mary had worked side by side with Rene, as an unpaid volunteer, for years. It was through Mary's efforts, both before Rene's death in 1978 and after, that the Essiac story remained alive.

To say that living history entered the room upon Mary's appearance in the doorway is to entirely miss the point. Mary McPherson is not merely the keeper of a flame, she is the flame in her own right. Anyone trying to put out the fire that Essiac lit in the lives of so many cancer sufferers would have a hard time dousing the enthusiasm Mary unfailingly projects not only about Essiac itself but about her lifelong friend Rene Caisse.

That the effort has on occasion left her feeling very alone is an inescapable conclusion anyone hearing her talk of Essiac must reach. She has talked to thousands about Essiac — doctors, lawyers, movie producers, government agencies, entrepreneurs, con artists, sales representatives, politicians— interested parties from as far away as Taiwan. She has seen them all. It was understandable then that when we met she was skeptical. I couldn't blame her. But her dedication to Essiac surfaced quickly, like a silken thread, and drew the patchwork of multiple purposes present in the room into a fine weave.

Lest one mistake Mary McPherson for a gentle granny always warm and kind to visitors, it must be said, she has a vibrant intellect, a finely honed gift of discernment, a steel trap insistence on accuracy. She knows what you intend to say before you say it, having heard it all before, and was more intimidating in the flesh than ever she had been when I was previously moving about Bracebridge and repeatedly hearing her name.

When invited to have 'the last word' in this rendering she instantly insisted that Rene herself should and would have 'the last word'.

Understandably, I had mistaken her for a nurse who aligned herself with Rene's cause. Mary quickly corrected the assumption, noting that she was not a nurse, that she had volunteered her time at Rene's side over the years; she then qualified why it was that she took no pay for her services by making this most emphatic statement about Rene Caisse: "She saved my husband and my mother from death by cancer and that was pay enough for me."

The defining moment of the meeting with Mary McPherson came when a quote from a doctor of years ago was repeated, that Rene Caisse perhaps had 'healing hands'. To this Mary answered with lightening swiftness and total confidence, and in doing so, emphatically gave Rene Caisse the last word: "Rene saved the lives of hundreds she had never met once in her life."

Yes, I was intimidated by Mary McPherson. I remain so. Should I ever have the pleasure of meeting her again, I will take nothing for granted. For, life remains a patchwork, and though I don't understand quilt making, I know quilts keep you warm. But most of all, I know when I have seen the finest silk.

SOURCES

PART I: *ACTS OF FAITH*

Chapter One : The Endtimers
1: William Carleton Gibson, The Canadians, Part II, Science and Medicine, Toronto, MacMillan Co. of Canada, Ltd. 1967

Chapter Two : An Ancient Dragon
1: William Carleton Gibson, The Canadians, Part II, Science and Medicine, Toronto, MacMillan Co. of Canada, Ltd. 1967
2: Bracebridge Examiner, Rene Caisse's Own Story
3: William Carleton Gibson, The Canadians, Part II, Science and Medicine, Toronto, MacMillan Co. of Canada, Ltd. 1967

Chapter Three: Unsung Aria
1. Dr. Leo Roy, Mastery Over Cancer, Westbank, British Columbia, 1988

Chapter Four: Nocturne In Pain and Suffering
1: Chronicle of Canada, Montreal, Chronicle Publications, 1990.
2: Rene Caisse, I Was Canada's Cancer Nurse: the Story of Essiac. Toronto. The Cancer Club of Toronto, 1980.
3: Snow & Allen, Homemakers Magazine, Could Essiac Halt Cancer? 1977, p.5.
4: Ibid.

Chapter Five: Through Irish Lace
1: Rene Caisse, I Was Canada's Cancer Nurse: the Story of Essiac. Toronto. The Cancer Club of Toronto, 1980.
2: Bernard Malamud, The Fixer, New York, Dell Publishing, 1966..
3: Matt: 13:57.

Chapter Six: A Prophet and A Lion.
1: Roy Greenway, Toronto Star.
2: Bracebridge Examiner, Rene Caisse Own's Story, Ted Britton, Editor. 1978.

Chapter Seven: Cross The Bridge And Turn Left
1: Dr. Leo Roy, Mastery Over Cancer, Westbank, British Columbia, 1988, p. 58
2: Ibid, p.61
3: Rene Caisse, I Was Canada's Cancer Nurse: the Story of Essiac. Toronto. The Cancer Club of Toronto, 1980.
4: Ibid.
5: Dr. Leo Roy, Mastery Over Cancer, Westbank, British Columbia, 1988, p. 58
6: Ibid, p.59
7: Ibid, p.33
8: Ibid, p.61
9: Ibid, p.59
10: Ibid, p.32
11:Rene Caisse, I Was Canada's Cancer Nurse: the Story of Essiac. Toronto. The Cancer

Club of Toronto, 1980.
12: Dr. Leo Roy, Mastery Over Cancer, Westbank, British Columbia, 1988, p, 58
13: Ibid, p.61
14: Ibid, p.82
15: Ibid, p.16
16: Ibid, p.25
17: Ibid, p.59
18: Ibid, p.69
19: Ibid, p.25
20: Ibid, p.82
21: Ibid, p.38
22: Ibid, p.51
23: Ibid, p.83
24: Ibid, p.45
25: Ibid, p.38
26: Ibid, p.61
27: Ibid, p.53
28: Ibid, p.39
29: Ibid, p.81
30: Ibid, p.75
31: Ibid, p.72
32: Ibid, p. 85
33: Ibid, p. 81
34: Ibid, p. 82
35: Ibid, p. 57
36: Ibid, p. 44
37: Ibid, p. 67
38: Ibid, p. 87
39: Ibid, p. 80
40: Ibid, p. 80
41: Ibid, p.63

Chapter Eight: The Art Of Healing
1: Dr. Leo Roy, Mastery Over Cancer, Westbank, British Columbia, 1988, p. 59
2: Ibid, p. 66
3: Ibid, p. 66
4: Ibid, p. 66
5: Ibid, p. 63
6: Bracebridge Examiner, Rene Caisse's Own Story
7: Rene Caisse, I Was Canada's Cancer Nurse: the Story of Essiac. Toronto. The Cancer Club of Toronto, 1980.
8: Ibid.

PART II: *ACTS OF HOPE*

Chapter One: The Politics of Persistence.
1: Snow & Allen, Homemakers Magazine, Could Essiac Halt Cancer? 1977. P.9, quoting Dr. Emma Carson
2: Dr. Guyatt, Curator and Instructor of Anatomy, University of Toronto, Letter to Rene Caisse for publication.
3: Ibid
4: Ibid.
5: Ibid.
6: Norman Cousins, The Healing Heart quoting Dr. Bernard Lown, M.D. Professor of

SOURCES

Cardiology, Harvard University, School of Public Health
7: Snow & Allen, Homemakers Magazine, Could Essiac Halt Cancer? 1977. p.10
8: Ibid, p. 10
9: Ibid, p. 10
10:Ibid, p. 9

Chapter two: When Owls Get The Vote
1: Michael Trent, song lyric, Spider In My Mailbox, c1996.
2: Bracebridge Examiner, Rene Caisse's Own Story, Part VIII, IX
3: Ibid.

Chapter Three: The 'Forever' Nurse.
1: Snow & Allen, Homemakers Magazine, Could Essiac Halt Cancer? 1977. p. 11
2: Bracebridge Examiner, Rene Caisse's Story, Part VIII, IX
3: Dr. Guyatt, Letter to Rene Caisse for publication.
4:S. Snow & Allen, Homemakers Magazine, Could Essiac Halt Cancer? 1977.
5: Ibid, p.13
6: Ibid.
7: Ibid.
8: Ibid.
9: Bracebridge Examiner, Rene Caisse's Own Story, Part VIII, IX

PART III: *A SINGULAR ACT OF CHARITY*

Chapter One: The Green Eyed Monster
1: Bracebridge Examiner, Rene Caisse's Own Story
2; Ibid, Part II

Chapter Three: Yesterday
1: Thomas Boon, 1963, of MacDonough, 1888, quoted by Lein, L.M. in Museum Musings, Nipigon, Ontario, April 9, 1974
2: Rene Caisse, I Was Canada's Cancer Nurse: the Story of Essiac. Toronto. The Cancer Club of Toronto, 1980.
3: Ibid.
4: Ibid.
5: Barry Lines, Cancer Cure That Worked!, Fifty years of Suppression, Marcus Books.
6: Resperin Canada, Rene M. Caisse Cancer Research Canada.
7: S. Snow, The Essence of Essiac, p.64
8: Barry Lines, Cancer Cure That Worked!, Fifty years of Suppression, Marcus Books quoted in Omni, February, 1993.
9: S. Snow, The Essence of Essiac, (Port Carling, ON: The Author) 1988, p. 57.
10: Ibid p.57.
11: Ibid p.58/59
12: Bracebridge Examiner, Rene Caisse's Own Story, Part XV
13: S. Snow, The Essence of Essiac, (Port Carling, ON: The Author) 1988, p.66
14: Rene Caisse, I Was Canada's Cancer Nurse: the Story of Essiac. Toronto. The Cancer Club of Toronto, 1980.
15: Ibid
16: Ibid
17: Ibid
18: National Center for Health Statistics.
19: Bracebridge Examiner, Rene Caisse's Own Story.
20: Barry Lines, Dr., Cancer Cure That Worked! Marcus Books.

INDEX OF ILLUSTRATIONS

Page A: Manitoba Street, mid-1890's, photographer unknown, courtesy Ken Veitch Collection.
Page B: The steamer 'Island', May 14, 1914, first year of the First World War. John Boyd Collection, National Archives of Canada, PA-061042
Page C: 1: Frizelda Caisse, Mary McPherson Collection, Bracebridge Library
2: Joseph Caisse, Mary McPherson Collection, Bracebridge Library
Page D: Rene Caisse, Mary McPherson Collection, Bracebridge Library
Page E: 1: British Lion Hotel, Nicholas Roche Collection, Lee Building, Bracebridge.
2: Lee Building, Photo by Paul Bennett, Rene M. Caisse Cancer Research Canada Collection, Ottawa.
3: Lee Building Plaque, Photo by Paul Bennett, Rene M. Caisse Cancer Research Canada Collection, Ottawa.
Page F: 1: Rene in Doorway, Mary McPherson Collection, Bracebridge Library.
2: Rene on clinic steps, Mary McPherson Collection, Bracebridge Library.
3: 1937 Announcement, Mary McPherson Collection, Bracebridge Library.
Page G: Dr. Frederick Banting, Photo by Arthur S. Goss, Oskar Klotz Collection, National Archives of Canada, PA-123481
Page H: 1: Queen's Park: Ontario Parliament Buildings, Toronto, Ontario, Albertyne Collection, National Archives of Canada, PA-032107
2: Premier Mitchel Hepburn, Premier of Ontario, Dr. Herbert L. Bruce, Lt. Gov. of Ontario, 1930's, Canadian Broadcasting Corporation Collection, National Archives, C-019531
Page I: Letter of Leslie Frost, Bracebridge Library.
Page J: Council Minutes, 1934, Bracebridge Library.
Page K: Evita Peron acknowledging cheers of crowd, Buenos Aires, Argentina, Sept. 1947, Photo by Michel Rougier, National Archives of Canada, PA-115278
Page L: Rene's last birthday: Mary McPherson Collection, Bracebridge Library
Page M: 1: Hiram Street House: Photo by Paul Bennett, Rene M. Caisse Cancer Research Canada Collection, Ottawa.
2: Pauline McGibbon, Lt. Governor of Ontario, Photo by Harry E. Palmer, National Archives of Canada PA-182395
Page N: Mary McPherson, T.P. Maloney attending City Council June, 2000. Photo by Paul Bennett, Rene M. Caisse Cancer Research Canada Collection, Ottawa.
Page O: Headstones of Rene, Frizelda, Joseph, Photo by Paul Bennett, Rene M. Caisse Cancer Research Canada Collection, Ottawa.
Page P: The bridge, Photo by Paul Bennett, Rene M. Caisse Cancer Research Canada Collection, Ottawa.
Page Q: Bronze memorial on granite base with plaque of Totem Pole Park, Bracebridge, Ontario, unveiled by Mayor Scott Northmore November 15, 2000.